THIS TRAINING DIARY BELONGS TO:

CONTACT NUMBER:

CONTACT EMAIL:

START DATE:

MY FITNESS GOALS:

	TARGET DATE / TIMESCALE
1.	
2.	
3.	
4.	
5.	
6.	
7.	

MY MEASUREMENTS:

	DATE:	DATE:	DATE:
HEIGHT			
WEIGHT			
BMI			
BODY FAT %			
WAIST			
HIPS			
RIGHT THIGH			
LEFT THIGH			
RIGHT CALF			
LEFT CALF			
R. UPPER ARM			
L. UPPER ARM			
CHEST			

MY PERSONAL BESTS:

EXERCISE:	DATE:	DATE:	DATE:
BACK SQUAT			
FRONT SQUAT			
DEADLIFT			
BENCH PRESS			

PROGRAMME OVERVIEW:

TRAINING PERIOD / BLOCK:

	SESSION PLAN
MON	
TUE	
WED	
THU	
FRI	
SAT	
SUN	

PROGRAMME OVERVIEW:

TRAINING PERIOD / BLOCK:

	SESSION PLAN
MON	
TUE	
WED	
THU	
FRI	
SAT	
SUN	

PROGRAMME OVERVIEW:

TRAINING PERIOD / BLOCK:

	SESSION PLAN
MON	
TUE	
WED	
THU	
FRI	
SAT	
SUN	

PROGRAMME OVERVIEW:

TRAINING PERIOD / BLOCK:

	SESSION PLAN
MON	
TUE	
WED	
THU	
FRI	
SAT	
SUN	
TRAINING PERIOD / BLOCK:	

PROGRAMME OVERVIEW:

TRAINING PERIOD / BLOCK:

	SESSION PLAN
MON	
TUE	
WED	
THU	
FRI	
SAT	
SUN	

PROGRAMME OVERVIEW:

TRAINING PERIOD / BLOCK:

	SESSION PLAN
MON	
TUE	
WED	
THU	
FRI	
SAT	
SUN	

PROGRAMME OVERVIEW:

TRAINING PERIOD / BLOCK:

	SESSION PLAN
MON	
TUE	
WED	
THU	
FRI	
SAT	
SUN	

PROGRAMME OVERVIEW:

TRAINING PERIOD / BLOCK:

	SESSION PLAN
MON	
TUE	
WED	
THU	
FRI	
SAT	
SUN	

PROGRAMME OVERVIEW:

TRAINING PERIOD / BLOCK:

	SESSION PLAN
MON	
TUE	
WED	
THU	
FRI	
SAT	
SUN	

PROGRAMME OVERVIEW:

TRAINING PERIOD / BLOCK:

	SESSION PLAN
MON	
TUE	
WED	
THU	
FRI	
SAT	
SUN	

PROGRAMME OVERVIEW:

TRAINING PERIOD / BLOCK:

	SESSION PLAN
MON	
TUE	
WED	
THU	
FRI	
SAT	
SUN	

PROGRAMME OVERVIEW:

<table>
<tr><td colspan="2">TRAINING PERIOD / BLOCK:</td></tr>
</table>

	SESSION PLAN
MON	
TUE	
WED	
THU	
FRI	
SAT	
SUN	

SESSION LOGBOOK

MON	TUE	WED	THU	FRI	SAT	SUN

Date:	Start Time:	Finish Time:

Session Name / Type:

STRENGTH & CONDITIONING

EXERCISE	SET 1	SET 2	SET 3	SET 4	SET 5
	REPS	REPS	REPS	REPS	REPS
	LOAD	LOAD	LOAD	LOAD	LOAD
	REPS	REPS	REPS	REPS	REPS
	LOAD	LOAD	LOAD	LOAD	LOAD
	REPS	REPS	REPS	REPS	REPS
	LOAD	LOAD	LOAD	LOAD	LOAD
	REPS	REPS	REPS	REPS	REPS
	LOAD	LOAD	LOAD	LOAD	LOAD
	REPS	REPS	REPS	REPS	REPS
	LOAD	LOAD	LOAD	LOAD	LOAD
	REPS	REPS	REPS	REPS	REPS
	LOAD	LOAD	LOAD	LOAD	LOAD
	REPS	REPS	REPS	REPS	REPS
	LOAD	LOAD	LOAD	LOAD	LOAD
	REPS	REPS	REPS	REPS	REPS
	LOAD	LOAD	LOAD	LOAD	LOAD
	REPS	REPS	REPS	REPS	REPS
	LOAD	LOAD	LOAD	LOAD	LOAD
	REPS	REPS	REPS	REPS	REPS
	LOAD	LOAD	LOAD	LOAD	LOAD

CARDIO

NAME / TYPE:				
TIME	**LEVEL**	**DISTANCE**	**HEART RATE**	**CALORIES**

NAME / TYPE:				
TIME	**LEVEL**	**DISTANCE**	**HEART RATE**	**CALORIES**

NOTES / OTHER

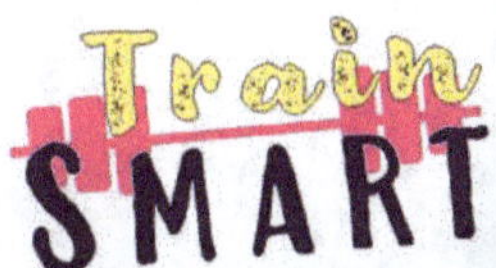

SESSION LOGBOOK

MON	TUE	WED	THU	FRI	SAT	SUN

Date:	Start Time:	Finish Time:

Session Name / Type:

STRENGTH & CONDITIONING

EXERCISE	SET 1	SET 2	SET 3	SET 4	SET 5
	REPS	REPS	REPS	REPS	REPS
	LOAD	LOAD	LOAD	LOAD	LOAD
	REPS	REPS	REPS	REPS	REPS
	LOAD	LOAD	LOAD	LOAD	LOAD
	REPS	REPS	REPS	REPS	REPS
	LOAD	LOAD	LOAD	LOAD	LOAD
	REPS	REPS	REPS	REPS	REPS
	LOAD	LOAD	LOAD	LOAD	LOAD
	REPS	REPS	REPS	REPS	REPS
	LOAD	LOAD	LOAD	LOAD	LOAD
	REPS	REPS	REPS	REPS	REPS
	LOAD	LOAD	LOAD	LOAD	LOAD
	REPS	REPS	REPS	REPS	REPS
	LOAD	LOAD	LOAD	LOAD	LOAD
	REPS	REPS	REPS	REPS	REPS
	LOAD	LOAD	LOAD	LOAD	LOAD
	REPS	REPS	REPS	REPS	REPS
	LOAD	LOAD	LOAD	LOAD	LOAD
	REPS	REPS	REPS	REPS	REPS
	LOAD	LOAD	LOAD	LOAD	LOAD

CARDIO

NAME / TYPE:				
TIME	**LEVEL**	**DISTANCE**	**HEART RATE**	**CALORIES**

NAME / TYPE:				
TIME	**LEVEL**	**DISTANCE**	**HEART RATE**	**CALORIES**

NOTES / OTHER

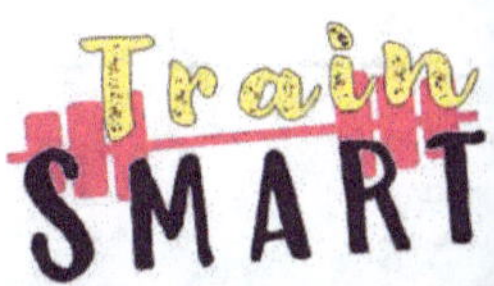

SESSION LOGBOOK

MON	TUE	WED	THU	FRI	SAT	SUN

Date:	Start Time:	Finish Time:

Session Name / Type:

STRENGTH & CONDITIONING

EXERCISE	SET 1	SET 2	SET 3	SET 4	SET 5
	REPS	REPS	REPS	REPS	REPS
	LOAD	LOAD	LOAD	LOAD	LOAD
	REPS	REPS	REPS	REPS	REPS
	LOAD	LOAD	LOAD	LOAD	LOAD
	REPS	REPS	REPS	REPS	REPS
	LOAD	LOAD	LOAD	LOAD	LOAD
	REPS	REPS	REPS	REPS	REPS
	LOAD	LOAD	LOAD	LOAD	LOAD
	REPS	REPS	REPS	REPS	REPS
	LOAD	LOAD	LOAD	LOAD	LOAD
	REPS	REPS	REPS	REPS	REPS
	LOAD	LOAD	LOAD	LOAD	LOAD
	REPS	REPS	REPS	REPS	REPS
	LOAD	LOAD	LOAD	LOAD	LOAD
	REPS	REPS	REPS	REPS	REPS
	LOAD	LOAD	LOAD	LOAD	LOAD
	REPS	REPS	REPS	REPS	REPS
	LOAD	LOAD	LOAD	LOAD	LOAD
	REPS	REPS	REPS	REPS	REPS
	LOAD	LOAD	LOAD	LOAD	LOAD

CARDIO

NAME / TYPE:				
TIME	LEVEL	DISTANCE	HEART RATE	CALORIES

NAME / TYPE:				
TIME	LEVEL	DISTANCE	HEART RATE	CALORIES

NOTES / OTHER

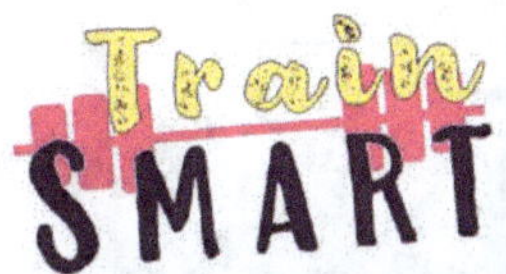

SESSION LOGBOOK

MON	TUE	WED	THU	FRI	SAT	SUN

Date:	Start Time:	Finish Time:

Session Name / Type:

STRENGTH & CONDITIONING

EXERCISE	SET 1	SET 2	SET 3	SET 4	SET 5
	REPS	REPS	REPS	REPS	REPS
	LOAD	LOAD	LOAD	LOAD	LOAD
	REPS	REPS	REPS	REPS	REPS
	LOAD	LOAD	LOAD	LOAD	LOAD
	REPS	REPS	REPS	REPS	REPS
	LOAD	LOAD	LOAD	LOAD	LOAD
	REPS	REPS	REPS	REPS	REPS
	LOAD	LOAD	LOAD	LOAD	LOAD
	REPS	REPS	REPS	REPS	REPS
	LOAD	LOAD	LOAD	LOAD	LOAD
	REPS	REPS	REPS	REPS	REPS
	LOAD	LOAD	LOAD	LOAD	LOAD
	REPS	REPS	REPS	REPS	REPS
	LOAD	LOAD	LOAD	LOAD	LOAD
	REPS	REPS	REPS	REPS	REPS
	LOAD	LOAD	LOAD	LOAD	LOAD
	REPS	REPS	REPS	REPS	REPS
	LOAD	LOAD	LOAD	LOAD	LOAD
	REPS	REPS	REPS	REPS	REPS
	LOAD	LOAD	LOAD	LOAD	LOAD

CARDIO

NAME / TYPE:				
TIME	**LEVEL**	**DISTANCE**	**HEART RATE**	**CALORIES**

NAME / TYPE:				
TIME	**LEVEL**	**DISTANCE**	**HEART RATE**	**CALORIES**

NOTES / OTHER

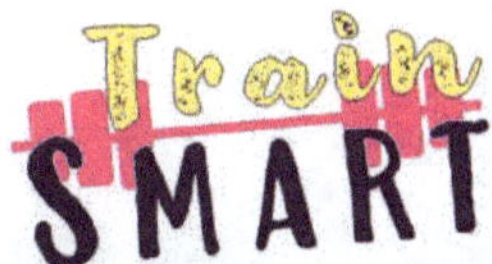

SESSION LOGBOOK

MON	TUE	WED	THU	FRI	SAT	SUN

Date:	Start Time:	Finish Time:

Session Name / Type:

STRENGTH & CONDITIONING

EXERCISE	SET 1	SET 2	SET 3	SET 4	SET 5
	REPS	REPS	REPS	REPS	REPS
	LOAD	LOAD	LOAD	LOAD	LOAD
	REPS	REPS	REPS	REPS	REPS
	LOAD	LOAD	LOAD	LOAD	LOAD
	REPS	REPS	REPS	REPS	REPS
	LOAD	LOAD	LOAD	LOAD	LOAD
	REPS	REPS	REPS	REPS	REPS
	LOAD	LOAD	LOAD	LOAD	LOAD
	REPS	REPS	REPS	REPS	REPS
	LOAD	LOAD	LOAD	LOAD	LOAD
	REPS	REPS	REPS	REPS	REPS
	LOAD	LOAD	LOAD	LOAD	LOAD
	REPS	REPS	REPS	REPS	REPS
	LOAD	LOAD	LOAD	LOAD	LOAD
	REPS	REPS	REPS	REPS	REPS
	LOAD	LOAD	LOAD	LOAD	LOAD
	REPS	REPS	REPS	REPS	REPS
	LOAD	LOAD	LOAD	LOAD	LOAD
	REPS	REPS	REPS	REPS	REPS
	LOAD	LOAD	LOAD	LOAD	LOAD

CARDIO

NAME / TYPE:				
TIME	LEVEL	DISTANCE	HEART RATE	CALORIES

NAME / TYPE:				
TIME	LEVEL	DISTANCE	HEART RATE	CALORIES

NOTES / OTHER

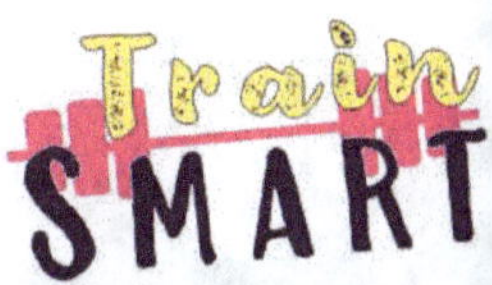

SESSION LOGBOOK

MON	TUE	WED	THU	FRI	SAT	SUN

Date:	Start Time:	Finish Time:

Session Name / Type:

STRENGTH & CONDITIONING

EXERCISE	SET 1	SET 2	SET 3	SET 4	SET 5
	REPS	REPS	REPS	REPS	REPS
	LOAD	LOAD	LOAD	LOAD	LOAD
	REPS	REPS	REPS	REPS	REPS
	LOAD	LOAD	LOAD	LOAD	LOAD
	REPS	REPS	REPS	REPS	REPS
	LOAD	LOAD	LOAD	LOAD	LOAD
	REPS	REPS	REPS	REPS	REPS
	LOAD	LOAD	LOAD	LOAD	LOAD
	REPS	REPS	REPS	REPS	REPS
	LOAD	LOAD	LOAD	LOAD	LOAD
	REPS	REPS	REPS	REPS	REPS
	LOAD	LOAD	LOAD	LOAD	LOAD
	REPS	REPS	REPS	REPS	REPS
	LOAD	LOAD	LOAD	LOAD	LOAD
	REPS	REPS	REPS	REPS	REPS
	LOAD	LOAD	LOAD	LOAD	LOAD
	REPS	REPS	REPS	REPS	REPS
	LOAD	LOAD	LOAD	LOAD	LOAD
	REPS	REPS	REPS	REPS	REPS
	LOAD	LOAD	LOAD	LOAD	LOAD

CARDIO

NAME / TYPE:				
TIME	LEVEL	DISTANCE	HEART RATE	CALORIES

NAME / TYPE:				
TIME	LEVEL	DISTANCE	HEART RATE	CALORIES

NOTES / OTHER

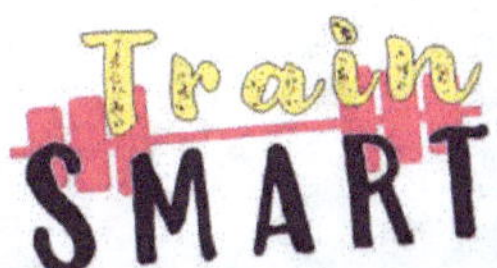

SESSION LOGBOOK

MON	TUE	WED	THU	FRI	SAT	SUN

Date:	Start Time:	Finish Time:

Session Name / Type:

STRENGTH & CONDITIONING

EXERCISE	SET 1	SET 2	SET 3	SET 4	SET 5
	REPS	REPS	REPS	REPS	REPS
	LOAD	LOAD	LOAD	LOAD	LOAD
	REPS	REPS	REPS	REPS	REPS
	LOAD	LOAD	LOAD	LOAD	LOAD
	REPS	REPS	REPS	REPS	REPS
	LOAD	LOAD	LOAD	LOAD	LOAD
	REPS	REPS	REPS	REPS	REPS
	LOAD	LOAD	LOAD	LOAD	LOAD
	REPS	REPS	REPS	REPS	REPS
	LOAD	LOAD	LOAD	LOAD	LOAD
	REPS	REPS	REPS	REPS	REPS
	LOAD	LOAD	LOAD	LOAD	LOAD
	REPS	REPS	REPS	REPS	REPS
	LOAD	LOAD	LOAD	LOAD	LOAD
	REPS	REPS	REPS	REPS	REPS
	LOAD	LOAD	LOAD	LOAD	LOAD
	REPS	REPS	REPS	REPS	REPS
	LOAD	LOAD	LOAD	LOAD	LOAD
	REPS	REPS	REPS	REPS	REPS
	LOAD	LOAD	LOAD	LOAD	LOAD

CARDIO

NAME / TYPE:				
TIME	**LEVEL**	**DISTANCE**	**HEART RATE**	**CALORIES**

NAME / TYPE:				
TIME	**LEVEL**	**DISTANCE**	**HEART RATE**	**CALORIES**

NOTES / OTHER

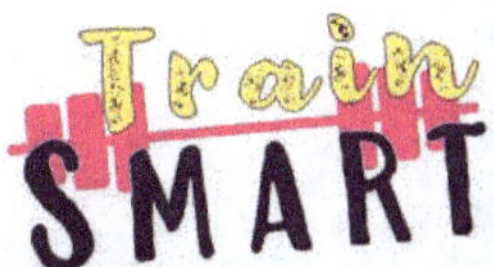

SESSION LOGBOOK

MON	TUE	WED	THU	FRI	SAT	SUN

Date: **Start Time:**   **Finish Time:**

Session Name / Type:

STRENGTH & CONDITIONING

EXERCISE	SET 1	SET 2	SET 3	SET 4	SET 5
	REPS LOAD	REPS LOAD	REPS LOAD	REPS LOAD	REPS LOAD
	REPS LOAD	REPS LOAD	REPS LOAD	REPS LOAD	REPS LOAD
	REPS LOAD	REPS LOAD	REPS LOAD	REPS LOAD	REPS LOAD
	REPS LOAD	REPS LOAD	REPS LOAD	REPS LOAD	REPS LOAD
	REPS LOAD	REPS LOAD	REPS LOAD	REPS LOAD	REPS LOAD
	REPS LOAD	REPS LOAD	REPS LOAD	REPS LOAD	REPS LOAD
	REPS LOAD	REPS LOAD	REPS LOAD	REPS LOAD	REPS LOAD
	REPS LOAD	REPS LOAD	REPS LOAD	REPS LOAD	REPS LOAD
	REPS LOAD	REPS LOAD	REPS LOAD	REPS LOAD	REPS LOAD
	REPS LOAD	REPS LOAD	REPS LOAD	REPS LOAD	REPS LOAD

CARDIO

NAME / TYPE:				
TIME	**LEVEL**	**DISTANCE**	**HEART RATE**	**CALORIES**

NAME / TYPE:				
TIME	**LEVEL**	**DISTANCE**	**HEART RATE**	**CALORIES**

NOTES / OTHER

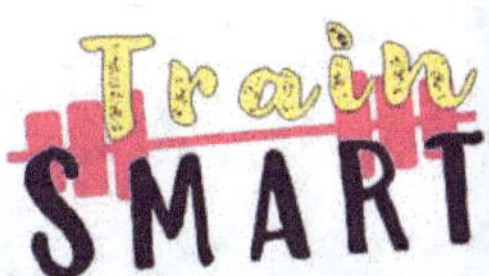

SESSION LOGBOOK

MON	TUE	WED	THU	FRI	SAT	SUN

Date:	Start Time:	Finish Time:

Session Name / Type:

STRENGTH & CONDITIONING

EXERCISE	SET 1	SET 2	SET 3	SET 4	SET 5
	REPS	REPS	REPS	REPS	REPS
	LOAD	LOAD	LOAD	LOAD	LOAD
	REPS	REPS	REPS	REPS	REPS
	LOAD	LOAD	LOAD	LOAD	LOAD
	REPS	REPS	REPS	REPS	REPS
	LOAD	LOAD	LOAD	LOAD	LOAD
	REPS	REPS	REPS	REPS	REPS
	LOAD	LOAD	LOAD	LOAD	LOAD
	REPS	REPS	REPS	REPS	REPS
	LOAD	LOAD	LOAD	LOAD	LOAD
	REPS	REPS	REPS	REPS	REPS
	LOAD	LOAD	LOAD	LOAD	LOAD
	REPS	REPS	REPS	REPS	REPS
	LOAD	LOAD	LOAD	LOAD	LOAD
	REPS	REPS	REPS	REPS	REPS
	LOAD	LOAD	LOAD	LOAD	LOAD
	REPS	REPS	REPS	REPS	REPS
	LOAD	LOAD	LOAD	LOAD	LOAD
	REPS	REPS	REPS	REPS	REPS
	LOAD	LOAD	LOAD	LOAD	LOAD

CARDIO

NAME / TYPE:				
TIME	**LEVEL**	**DISTANCE**	**HEART RATE**	**CALORIES**

NAME / TYPE:				
TIME	**LEVEL**	**DISTANCE**	**HEART RATE**	**CALORIES**

NOTES / OTHER

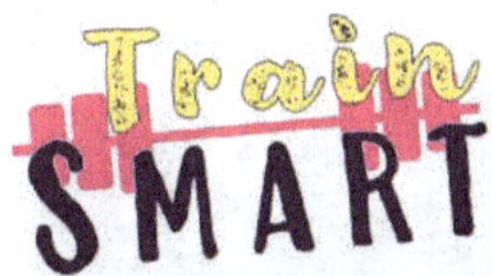

SESSION LOGBOOK

MON	TUE	WED	THU	FRI	SAT	SUN

Date:	Start Time:	Finish Time:

Session Name / Type:

STRENGTH & CONDITIONING

EXERCISE	SET 1	SET 2	SET 3	SET 4	SET 5
	REPS LOAD	REPS LOAD	REPS LOAD	REPS LOAD	REPS LOAD
	REPS LOAD	REPS LOAD	REPS LOAD	REPS LOAD	REPS LOAD
	REPS LOAD	REPS LOAD	REPS LOAD	REPS LOAD	REPS LOAD
	REPS LOAD	REPS LOAD	REPS LOAD	REPS LOAD	REPS LOAD
	REPS LOAD	REPS LOAD	REPS LOAD	REPS LOAD	REPS LOAD
	REPS LOAD	REPS LOAD	REPS LOAD	REPS LOAD	REPS LOAD
	REPS LOAD	REPS LOAD	REPS LOAD	REPS LOAD	REPS LOAD
	REPS LOAD	REPS LOAD	REPS LOAD	REPS LOAD	REPS LOAD
	REPS LOAD	REPS LOAD	REPS LOAD	REPS LOAD	REPS LOAD
	REPS LOAD	REPS LOAD	REPS LOAD	REPS LOAD	REPS LOAD

CARDIO

NAME / TYPE:				
TIME	**LEVEL**	**DISTANCE**	**HEART RATE**	**CALORIES**

NAME / TYPE:				
TIME	**LEVEL**	**DISTANCE**	**HEART RATE**	**CALORIES**

NOTES / OTHER

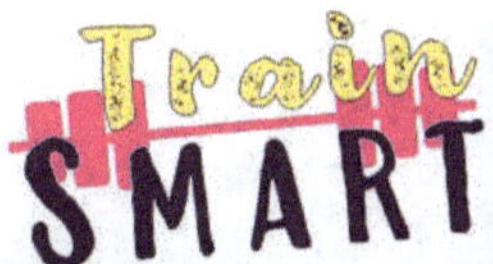

SESSION LOGBOOK

MON	TUE	WED	THU	FRI	SAT	SUN

Date:	Start Time:	Finish Time:

Session Name / Type:

STRENGTH & CONDITIONING

EXERCISE	SET 1	SET 2	SET 3	SET 4	SET 5
	REPS	REPS	REPS	REPS	REPS
	LOAD	LOAD	LOAD	LOAD	LOAD
	REPS	REPS	REPS	REPS	REPS
	LOAD	LOAD	LOAD	LOAD	LOAD
	REPS	REPS	REPS	REPS	REPS
	LOAD	LOAD	LOAD	LOAD	LOAD
	REPS	REPS	REPS	REPS	REPS
	LOAD	LOAD	LOAD	LOAD	LOAD
	REPS	REPS	REPS	REPS	REPS
	LOAD	LOAD	LOAD	LOAD	LOAD
	REPS	REPS	REPS	REPS	REPS
	LOAD	LOAD	LOAD	LOAD	LOAD
	REPS	REPS	REPS	REPS	REPS
	LOAD	LOAD	LOAD	LOAD	LOAD
	REPS	REPS	REPS	REPS	REPS
	LOAD	LOAD	LOAD	LOAD	LOAD
	REPS	REPS	REPS	REPS	REPS
	LOAD	LOAD	LOAD	LOAD	LOAD
	REPS	REPS	REPS	REPS	REPS
	LOAD	LOAD	LOAD	LOAD	LOAD

CARDIO

NAME / TYPE:				
TIME	LEVEL	DISTANCE	HEART RATE	CALORIES

NAME / TYPE:				
TIME	LEVEL	DISTANCE	HEART RATE	CALORIES

NOTES / OTHER

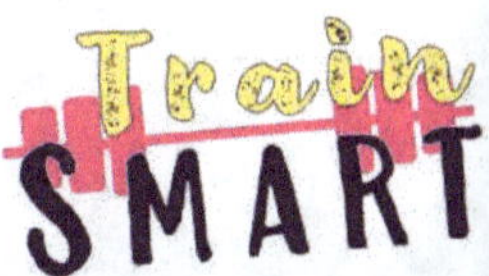

SESSION LOGBOOK

MON	TUE	WED	THU	FRI	SAT	SUN

Date:	Start Time:	Finish Time:

Session Name / Type:

STRENGTH & CONDITIONING

EXERCISE	SET 1	SET 2	SET 3	SET 4	SET 5
	REPS	REPS	REPS	REPS	REPS
	LOAD	LOAD	LOAD	LOAD	LOAD
	REPS	REPS	REPS	REPS	REPS
	LOAD	LOAD	LOAD	LOAD	LOAD
	REPS	REPS	REPS	REPS	REPS
	LOAD	LOAD	LOAD	LOAD	LOAD
	REPS	REPS	REPS	REPS	REPS
	LOAD	LOAD	LOAD	LOAD	LOAD
	REPS	REPS	REPS	REPS	REPS
	LOAD	LOAD	LOAD	LOAD	LOAD
	REPS	REPS	REPS	REPS	REPS
	LOAD	LOAD	LOAD	LOAD	LOAD
	REPS	REPS	REPS	REPS	REPS
	LOAD	LOAD	LOAD	LOAD	LOAD
	REPS	REPS	REPS	REPS	REPS
	LOAD	LOAD	LOAD	LOAD	LOAD
	REPS	REPS	REPS	REPS	REPS
	LOAD	LOAD	LOAD	LOAD	LOAD
	REPS	REPS	REPS	REPS	REPS
	LOAD	LOAD	LOAD	LOAD	LOAD

CARDIO

NAME / TYPE:				
TIME	**LEVEL**	**DISTANCE**	**HEART RATE**	**CALORIES**

NAME / TYPE:				
TIME	**LEVEL**	**DISTANCE**	**HEART RATE**	**CALORIES**

NOTES / OTHER

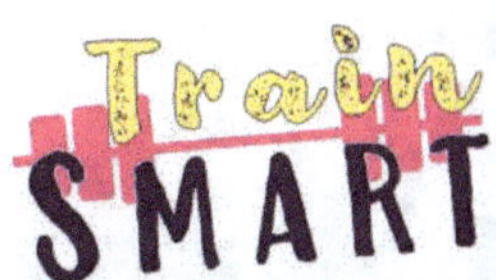

SESSION LOGBOOK

MON	TUE	WED	THU	FRI	SAT	SUN

Date:	Start Time:	Finish Time:

Session Name / Type:

STRENGTH & CONDITIONING

EXERCISE	SET 1	SET 2	SET 3	SET 4	SET 5
	REPS	REPS	REPS	REPS	REPS
	LOAD	LOAD	LOAD	LOAD	LOAD
	REPS	REPS	REPS	REPS	REPS
	LOAD	LOAD	LOAD	LOAD	LOAD
	REPS	REPS	REPS	REPS	REPS
	LOAD	LOAD	LOAD	LOAD	LOAD
	REPS	REPS	REPS	REPS	REPS
	LOAD	LOAD	LOAD	LOAD	LOAD
	REPS	REPS	REPS	REPS	REPS
	LOAD	LOAD	LOAD	LOAD	LOAD
	REPS	REPS	REPS	REPS	REPS
	LOAD	LOAD	LOAD	LOAD	LOAD
	REPS	REPS	REPS	REPS	REPS
	LOAD	LOAD	LOAD	LOAD	LOAD
	REPS	REPS	REPS	REPS	REPS
	LOAD	LOAD	LOAD	LOAD	LOAD
	REPS	REPS	REPS	REPS	REPS
	LOAD	LOAD	LOAD	LOAD	LOAD
	REPS	REPS	REPS	REPS	REPS
	LOAD	LOAD	LOAD	LOAD	LOAD

CARDIO

NAME / TYPE:				
TIME	**LEVEL**	**DISTANCE**	**HEART RATE**	**CALORIES**

NAME / TYPE:				
TIME	**LEVEL**	**DISTANCE**	**HEART RATE**	**CALORIES**

NOTES / OTHER

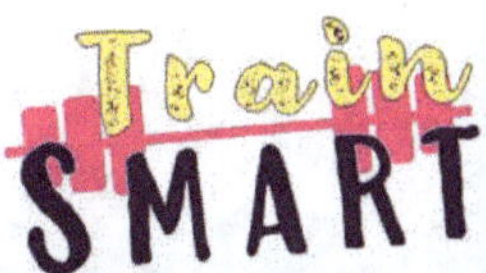

SESSION LOGBOOK

MON	TUE	WED	THU	FRI	SAT	SUN

Date:	Start Time:	Finish Time:

Session Name / Type:

STRENGTH & CONDITIONING

EXERCISE	SET 1	SET 2	SET 3	SET 4	SET 5
	REPS	REPS	REPS	REPS	REPS
	LOAD	LOAD	LOAD	LOAD	LOAD
	REPS	REPS	REPS	REPS	REPS
	LOAD	LOAD	LOAD	LOAD	LOAD
	REPS	REPS	REPS	REPS	REPS
	LOAD	LOAD	LOAD	LOAD	LOAD
	REPS	REPS	REPS	REPS	REPS
	LOAD	LOAD	LOAD	LOAD	LOAD
	REPS	REPS	REPS	REPS	REPS
	LOAD	LOAD	LOAD	LOAD	LOAD
	REPS	REPS	REPS	REPS	REPS
	LOAD	LOAD	LOAD	LOAD	LOAD
	REPS	REPS	REPS	REPS	REPS
	LOAD	LOAD	LOAD	LOAD	LOAD
	REPS	REPS	REPS	REPS	REPS
	LOAD	LOAD	LOAD	LOAD	LOAD
	REPS	REPS	REPS	REPS	REPS
	LOAD	LOAD	LOAD	LOAD	LOAD
	REPS	REPS	REPS	REPS	REPS
	LOAD	LOAD	LOAD	LOAD	LOAD

CARDIO

NAME / TYPE:				
TIME	**LEVEL**	**DISTANCE**	**HEART RATE**	**CALORIES**

NAME / TYPE:				
TIME	**LEVEL**	**DISTANCE**	**HEART RATE**	**CALORIES**

NOTES / OTHER

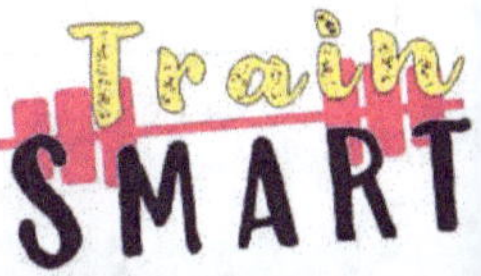

SESSION LOGBOOK

MON	TUE	WED	THU	FRI	SAT	SUN

Date:	Start Time:	Finish Time:

Session Name / Type:

STRENGTH & CONDITIONING

EXERCISE	SET 1	SET 2	SET 3	SET 4	SET 5
	REPS	REPS	REPS	REPS	REPS
	LOAD	LOAD	LOAD	LOAD	LOAD
	REPS	REPS	REPS	REPS	REPS
	LOAD	LOAD	LOAD	LOAD	LOAD
	REPS	REPS	REPS	REPS	REPS
	LOAD	LOAD	LOAD	LOAD	LOAD
	REPS	REPS	REPS	REPS	REPS
	LOAD	LOAD	LOAD	LOAD	LOAD
	REPS	REPS	REPS	REPS	REPS
	LOAD	LOAD	LOAD	LOAD	LOAD
	REPS	REPS	REPS	REPS	REPS
	LOAD	LOAD	LOAD	LOAD	LOAD
	REPS	REPS	REPS	REPS	REPS
	LOAD	LOAD	LOAD	LOAD	LOAD
	REPS	REPS	REPS	REPS	REPS
	LOAD	LOAD	LOAD	LOAD	LOAD
	REPS	REPS	REPS	REPS	REPS
	LOAD	LOAD	LOAD	LOAD	LOAD
	REPS	REPS	REPS	REPS	REPS
	LOAD	LOAD	LOAD	LOAD	LOAD

CARDIO

NAME / TYPE:				
TIME	**LEVEL**	**DISTANCE**	**HEART RATE**	**CALORIES**

NAME / TYPE:				
TIME	**LEVEL**	**DISTANCE**	**HEART RATE**	**CALORIES**

NOTES / OTHER

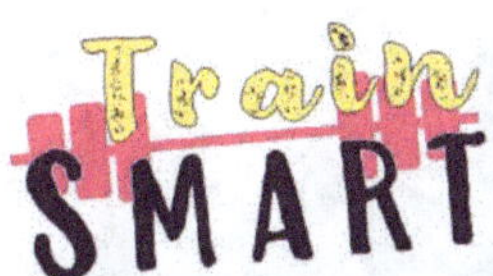

SESSION LOGBOOK

MON	TUE	WED	THU	FRI	SAT	SUN

Date:	Start Time:	Finish Time:

Session Name / Type:

STRENGTH & CONDITIONING

EXERCISE	SET 1	SET 2	SET 3	SET 4	SET 5
	REPS	REPS	REPS	REPS	REPS
	LOAD	LOAD	LOAD	LOAD	LOAD
	REPS	REPS	REPS	REPS	REPS
	LOAD	LOAD	LOAD	LOAD	LOAD
	REPS	REPS	REPS	REPS	REPS
	LOAD	LOAD	LOAD	LOAD	LOAD
	REPS	REPS	REPS	REPS	REPS
	LOAD	LOAD	LOAD	LOAD	LOAD
	REPS	REPS	REPS	REPS	REPS
	LOAD	LOAD	LOAD	LOAD	LOAD
	REPS	REPS	REPS	REPS	REPS
	LOAD	LOAD	LOAD	LOAD	LOAD
	REPS	REPS	REPS	REPS	REPS
	LOAD	LOAD	LOAD	LOAD	LOAD
	REPS	REPS	REPS	REPS	REPS
	LOAD	LOAD	LOAD	LOAD	LOAD
	REPS	REPS	REPS	REPS	REPS
	LOAD	LOAD	LOAD	LOAD	LOAD
	REPS	REPS	REPS	REPS	REPS
	LOAD	LOAD	LOAD	LOAD	LOAD

CARDIO

NAME / TYPE:				
TIME	**LEVEL**	**DISTANCE**	**HEART RATE**	**CALORIES**

NAME / TYPE:				
TIME	**LEVEL**	**DISTANCE**	**HEART RATE**	**CALORIES**

NOTES / OTHER

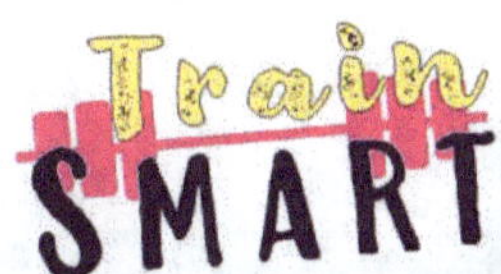

SESSION LOGBOOK

MON	TUE	WED	THU	FRI	SAT	SUN

Date:		Start Time:		Finish Time:	

Session Name / Type:

STRENGTH & CONDITIONING

EXERCISE	SET 1	SET 2	SET 3	SET 4	SET 5
	REPS	REPS	REPS	REPS	REPS
	LOAD	LOAD	LOAD	LOAD	LOAD
	REPS	REPS	REPS	REPS	REPS
	LOAD	LOAD	LOAD	LOAD	LOAD
	REPS	REPS	REPS	REPS	REPS
	LOAD	LOAD	LOAD	LOAD	LOAD
	REPS	REPS	REPS	REPS	REPS
	LOAD	LOAD	LOAD	LOAD	LOAD
	REPS	REPS	REPS	REPS	REPS
	LOAD	LOAD	LOAD	LOAD	LOAD
	REPS	REPS	REPS	REPS	REPS
	LOAD	LOAD	LOAD	LOAD	LOAD
	REPS	REPS	REPS	REPS	REPS
	LOAD	LOAD	LOAD	LOAD	LOAD
	REPS	REPS	REPS	REPS	REPS
	LOAD	LOAD	LOAD	LOAD	LOAD
	REPS	REPS	REPS	REPS	REPS
	LOAD	LOAD	LOAD	LOAD	LOAD
	REPS	REPS	REPS	REPS	REPS
	LOAD	LOAD	LOAD	LOAD	LOAD

CARDIO

NAME / TYPE:				
TIME	**LEVEL**	**DISTANCE**	**HEART RATE**	**CALORIES**

NAME / TYPE:				
TIME	**LEVEL**	**DISTANCE**	**HEART RATE**	**CALORIES**

NOTES / OTHER

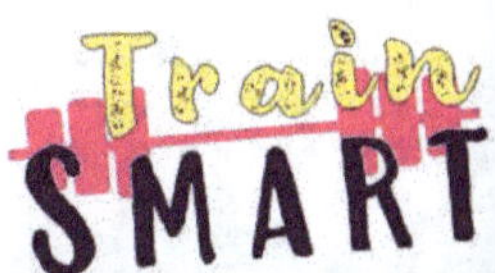

SESSION LOGBOOK

MON	TUE	WED	THU	FRI	SAT	SUN

Date:	Start Time:	Finish Time:

Session Name / Type:

STRENGTH & CONDITIONING

EXERCISE	SET 1	SET 2	SET 3	SET 4	SET 5
	REPS	REPS	REPS	REPS	REPS
	LOAD	LOAD	LOAD	LOAD	LOAD
	REPS	REPS	REPS	REPS	REPS
	LOAD	LOAD	LOAD	LOAD	LOAD
	REPS	REPS	REPS	REPS	REPS
	LOAD	LOAD	LOAD	LOAD	LOAD
	REPS	REPS	REPS	REPS	REPS
	LOAD	LOAD	LOAD	LOAD	LOAD
	REPS	REPS	REPS	REPS	REPS
	LOAD	LOAD	LOAD	LOAD	LOAD
	REPS	REPS	REPS	REPS	REPS
	LOAD	LOAD	LOAD	LOAD	LOAD
	REPS	REPS	REPS	REPS	REPS
	LOAD	LOAD	LOAD	LOAD	LOAD
	REPS	REPS	REPS	REPS	REPS
	LOAD	LOAD	LOAD	LOAD	LOAD
	REPS	REPS	REPS	REPS	REPS
	LOAD	LOAD	LOAD	LOAD	LOAD
	REPS	REPS	REPS	REPS	REPS
	LOAD	LOAD	LOAD	LOAD	LOAD

CARDIO

NAME / TYPE:				
TIME	**LEVEL**	**DISTANCE**	**HEART RATE**	**CALORIES**

NAME / TYPE:				
TIME	**LEVEL**	**DISTANCE**	**HEART RATE**	**CALORIES**

NOTES / OTHER

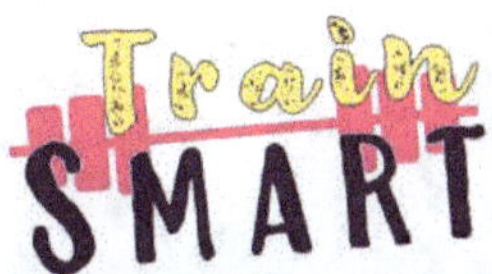

SESSION LOGBOOK

MON	TUE	WED	THU	FRI	SAT	SUN

Date:	Start Time:	Finish Time:

Session Name / Type:

STRENGTH & CONDITIONING

EXERCISE	SET 1	SET 2	SET 3	SET 4	SET 5
	REPS	REPS	REPS	REPS	REPS
	LOAD	LOAD	LOAD	LOAD	LOAD
	REPS	REPS	REPS	REPS	REPS
	LOAD	LOAD	LOAD	LOAD	LOAD
	REPS	REPS	REPS	REPS	REPS
	LOAD	LOAD	LOAD	LOAD	LOAD
	REPS	REPS	REPS	REPS	REPS
	LOAD	LOAD	LOAD	LOAD	LOAD
	REPS	REPS	REPS	REPS	REPS
	LOAD	LOAD	LOAD	LOAD	LOAD
	REPS	REPS	REPS	REPS	REPS
	LOAD	LOAD	LOAD	LOAD	LOAD
	REPS	REPS	REPS	REPS	REPS
	LOAD	LOAD	LOAD	LOAD	LOAD
	REPS	REPS	REPS	REPS	REPS
	LOAD	LOAD	LOAD	LOAD	LOAD
	REPS	REPS	REPS	REPS	REPS
	LOAD	LOAD	LOAD	LOAD	LOAD
	REPS	REPS	REPS	REPS	REPS
	LOAD	LOAD	LOAD	LOAD	LOAD

CARDIO

NAME / TYPE:				
TIME	**LEVEL**	**DISTANCE**	**HEART RATE**	**CALORIES**

NAME / TYPE:				
TIME	**LEVEL**	**DISTANCE**	**HEART RATE**	**CALORIES**

NOTES / OTHER

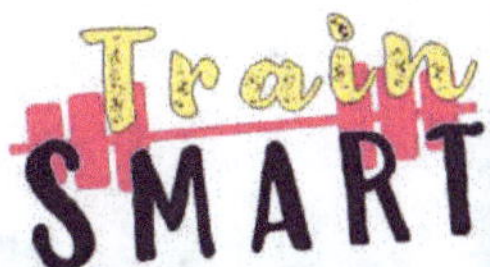

SESSION LOGBOOK

MON	TUE	WED	THU	FRI	SAT	SUN

Date:	Start Time:	Finish Time:

Session Name / Type:

STRENGTH & CONDITIONING

EXERCISE	SET 1	SET 2	SET 3	SET 4	SET 5
	REPS	REPS	REPS	REPS	REPS
	LOAD	LOAD	LOAD	LOAD	LOAD
	REPS	REPS	REPS	REPS	REPS
	LOAD	LOAD	LOAD	LOAD	LOAD
	REPS	REPS	REPS	REPS	REPS
	LOAD	LOAD	LOAD	LOAD	LOAD
	REPS	REPS	REPS	REPS	REPS
	LOAD	LOAD	LOAD	LOAD	LOAD
	REPS	REPS	REPS	REPS	REPS
	LOAD	LOAD	LOAD	LOAD	LOAD
	REPS	REPS	REPS	REPS	REPS
	LOAD	LOAD	LOAD	LOAD	LOAD
	REPS	REPS	REPS	REPS	REPS
	LOAD	LOAD	LOAD	LOAD	LOAD
	REPS	REPS	REPS	REPS	REPS
	LOAD	LOAD	LOAD	LOAD	LOAD
	REPS	REPS	REPS	REPS	REPS
	LOAD	LOAD	LOAD	LOAD	LOAD
	REPS	REPS	REPS	REPS	REPS
	LOAD	LOAD	LOAD	LOAD	LOAD

CARDIO

NAME / TYPE:				
TIME	**LEVEL**	**DISTANCE**	**HEART RATE**	**CALORIES**

NAME / TYPE:				
TIME	**LEVEL**	**DISTANCE**	**HEART RATE**	**CALORIES**

NOTES / OTHER

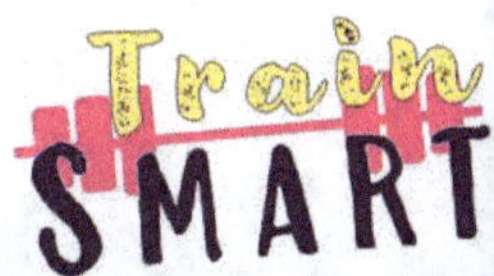

SESSION LOGBOOK

MON	TUE	WED	THU	FRI	SAT	SUN

Date:	Start Time:	Finish Time:

Session Name / Type:

STRENGTH & CONDITIONING

EXERCISE	SET 1	SET 2	SET 3	SET 4	SET 5
	REPS	REPS	REPS	REPS	REPS
	LOAD	LOAD	LOAD	LOAD	LOAD
	REPS	REPS	REPS	REPS	REPS
	LOAD	LOAD	LOAD	LOAD	LOAD
	REPS	REPS	REPS	REPS	REPS
	LOAD	LOAD	LOAD	LOAD	LOAD
	REPS	REPS	REPS	REPS	REPS
	LOAD	LOAD	LOAD	LOAD	LOAD
	REPS	REPS	REPS	REPS	REPS
	LOAD	LOAD	LOAD	LOAD	LOAD
	REPS	REPS	REPS	REPS	REPS
	LOAD	LOAD	LOAD	LOAD	LOAD
	REPS	REPS	REPS	REPS	REPS
	LOAD	LOAD	LOAD	LOAD	LOAD
	REPS	REPS	REPS	REPS	REPS
	LOAD	LOAD	LOAD	LOAD	LOAD
	REPS	REPS	REPS	REPS	REPS
	LOAD	LOAD	LOAD	LOAD	LOAD
	REPS	REPS	REPS	REPS	REPS
	LOAD	LOAD	LOAD	LOAD	LOAD

CARDIO

NAME / TYPE:				
TIME	**LEVEL**	**DISTANCE**	**HEART RATE**	**CALORIES**

NAME / TYPE:				
TIME	**LEVEL**	**DISTANCE**	**HEART RATE**	**CALORIES**

NOTES / OTHER

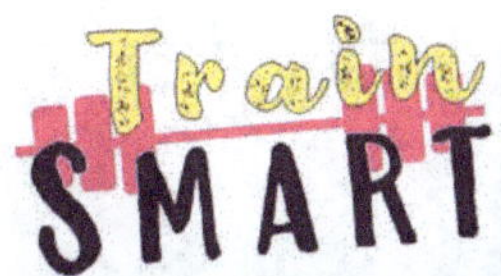

SESSION LOGBOOK

MON	TUE	WED	THU	FRI	SAT	SUN

Date:	Start Time:	Finish Time:

Session Name / Type:

STRENGTH & CONDITIONING

EXERCISE	SET 1	SET 2	SET 3	SET 4	SET 5
	REPS	REPS	REPS	REPS	REPS
	LOAD	LOAD	LOAD	LOAD	LOAD
	REPS	REPS	REPS	REPS	REPS
	LOAD	LOAD	LOAD	LOAD	LOAD
	REPS	REPS	REPS	REPS	REPS
	LOAD	LOAD	LOAD	LOAD	LOAD
	REPS	REPS	REPS	REPS	REPS
	LOAD	LOAD	LOAD	LOAD	LOAD
	REPS	REPS	REPS	REPS	REPS
	LOAD	LOAD	LOAD	LOAD	LOAD
	REPS	REPS	REPS	REPS	REPS
	LOAD	LOAD	LOAD	LOAD	LOAD
	REPS	REPS	REPS	REPS	REPS
	LOAD	LOAD	LOAD	LOAD	LOAD
	REPS	REPS	REPS	REPS	REPS
	LOAD	LOAD	LOAD	LOAD	LOAD
	REPS	REPS	REPS	REPS	REPS
	LOAD	LOAD	LOAD	LOAD	LOAD
	REPS	REPS	REPS	REPS	REPS
	LOAD	LOAD	LOAD	LOAD	LOAD

CARDIO

NAME / TYPE:				
TIME	**LEVEL**	**DISTANCE**	**HEART RATE**	**CALORIES**

NAME / TYPE:				
TIME	**LEVEL**	**DISTANCE**	**HEART RATE**	**CALORIES**

NOTES / OTHER

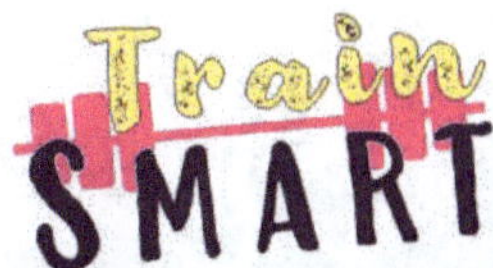

SESSION LOGBOOK

MON	TUE	WED	THU	FRI	SAT	SUN

Date:	Start Time:	Finish Time:

Session Name / Type:

STRENGTH & CONDITIONING

EXERCISE	SET 1	SET 2	SET 3	SET 4	SET 5
	REPS	REPS	REPS	REPS	REPS
	LOAD	LOAD	LOAD	LOAD	LOAD
	REPS	REPS	REPS	REPS	REPS
	LOAD	LOAD	LOAD	LOAD	LOAD
	REPS	REPS	REPS	REPS	REPS
	LOAD	LOAD	LOAD	LOAD	LOAD
	REPS	REPS	REPS	REPS	REPS
	LOAD	LOAD	LOAD	LOAD	LOAD
	REPS	REPS	REPS	REPS	REPS
	LOAD	LOAD	LOAD	LOAD	LOAD
	REPS	REPS	REPS	REPS	REPS
	LOAD	LOAD	LOAD	LOAD	LOAD
	REPS	REPS	REPS	REPS	REPS
	LOAD	LOAD	LOAD	LOAD	LOAD
	REPS	REPS	REPS	REPS	REPS
	LOAD	LOAD	LOAD	LOAD	LOAD
	REPS	REPS	REPS	REPS	REPS
	LOAD	LOAD	LOAD	LOAD	LOAD
	REPS	REPS	REPS	REPS	REPS
	LOAD	LOAD	LOAD	LOAD	LOAD

CARDIO

NAME / TYPE:				
TIME	**LEVEL**	**DISTANCE**	**HEART RATE**	**CALORIES**

NAME / TYPE:				
TIME	**LEVEL**	**DISTANCE**	**HEART RATE**	**CALORIES**

NOTES / OTHER

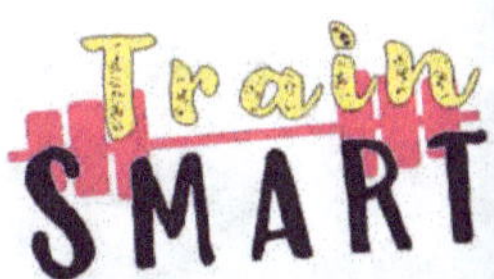

SESSION LOGBOOK

MON	TUE	WED	THU	FRI	SAT	SUN

Date:	Start Time:	Finish Time:

Session Name / Type:

STRENGTH & CONDITIONING

EXERCISE	SET 1	SET 2	SET 3	SET 4	SET 5
	REPS	REPS	REPS	REPS	REPS
	LOAD	LOAD	LOAD	LOAD	LOAD
	REPS	REPS	REPS	REPS	REPS
	LOAD	LOAD	LOAD	LOAD	LOAD
	REPS	REPS	REPS	REPS	REPS
	LOAD	LOAD	LOAD	LOAD	LOAD
	REPS	REPS	REPS	REPS	REPS
	LOAD	LOAD	LOAD	LOAD	LOAD
	REPS	REPS	REPS	REPS	REPS
	LOAD	LOAD	LOAD	LOAD	LOAD
	REPS	REPS	REPS	REPS	REPS
	LOAD	LOAD	LOAD	LOAD	LOAD
	REPS	REPS	REPS	REPS	REPS
	LOAD	LOAD	LOAD	LOAD	LOAD
	REPS	REPS	REPS	REPS	REPS
	LOAD	LOAD	LOAD	LOAD	LOAD
	REPS	REPS	REPS	REPS	REPS
	LOAD	LOAD	LOAD	LOAD	LOAD
	REPS	REPS	REPS	REPS	REPS
	LOAD	LOAD	LOAD	LOAD	LOAD

CARDIO

NAME / TYPE:				
TIME	**LEVEL**	**DISTANCE**	**HEART RATE**	**CALORIES**

NAME / TYPE:				
TIME	**LEVEL**	**DISTANCE**	**HEART RATE**	**CALORIES**

NOTES / OTHER

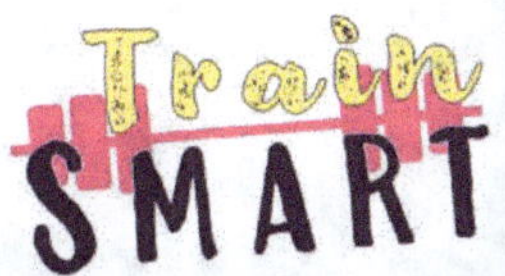

SESSION LOGBOOK

MON	TUE	WED	THU	FRI	SAT	SUN

Date:	Start Time:	Finish Time:

Session Name / Type:

STRENGTH & CONDITIONING

EXERCISE	SET 1	SET 2	SET 3	SET 4	SET 5
	REPS	REPS	REPS	REPS	REPS
	LOAD	LOAD	LOAD	LOAD	LOAD
	REPS	REPS	REPS	REPS	REPS
	LOAD	LOAD	LOAD	LOAD	LOAD
	REPS	REPS	REPS	REPS	REPS
	LOAD	LOAD	LOAD	LOAD	LOAD
	REPS	REPS	REPS	REPS	REPS
	LOAD	LOAD	LOAD	LOAD	LOAD
	REPS	REPS	REPS	REPS	REPS
	LOAD	LOAD	LOAD	LOAD	LOAD
	REPS	REPS	REPS	REPS	REPS
	LOAD	LOAD	LOAD	LOAD	LOAD
	REPS	REPS	REPS	REPS	REPS
	LOAD	LOAD	LOAD	LOAD	LOAD
	REPS	REPS	REPS	REPS	REPS
	LOAD	LOAD	LOAD	LOAD	LOAD
	REPS	REPS	REPS	REPS	REPS
	LOAD	LOAD	LOAD	LOAD	LOAD
	REPS	REPS	REPS	REPS	REPS
	LOAD	LOAD	LOAD	LOAD	LOAD

CARDIO

NAME / TYPE:				
TIME	**LEVEL**	**DISTANCE**	**HEART RATE**	**CALORIES**

NAME / TYPE:				
TIME	**LEVEL**	**DISTANCE**	**HEART RATE**	**CALORIES**

NOTES / OTHER

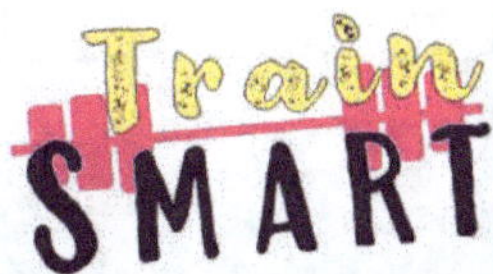

SESSION LOGBOOK

MON	TUE	WED	THU	FRI	SAT	SUN

Date:	Start Time:	Finish Time:

Session Name / Type:

STRENGTH & CONDITIONING

EXERCISE	SET 1	SET 2	SET 3	SET 4	SET 5
	REPS	REPS	REPS	REPS	REPS
	LOAD	LOAD	LOAD	LOAD	LOAD
	REPS	REPS	REPS	REPS	REPS
	LOAD	LOAD	LOAD	LOAD	LOAD
	REPS	REPS	REPS	REPS	REPS
	LOAD	LOAD	LOAD	LOAD	LOAD
	REPS	REPS	REPS	REPS	REPS
	LOAD	LOAD	LOAD	LOAD	LOAD
	REPS	REPS	REPS	REPS	REPS
	LOAD	LOAD	LOAD	LOAD	LOAD
	REPS	REPS	REPS	REPS	REPS
	LOAD	LOAD	LOAD	LOAD	LOAD
	REPS	REPS	REPS	REPS	REPS
	LOAD	LOAD	LOAD	LOAD	LOAD
	REPS	REPS	REPS	REPS	REPS
	LOAD	LOAD	LOAD	LOAD	LOAD
	REPS	REPS	REPS	REPS	REPS
	LOAD	LOAD	LOAD	LOAD	LOAD
	REPS	REPS	REPS	REPS	REPS
	LOAD	LOAD	LOAD	LOAD	LOAD

CARDIO

NAME / TYPE:				
TIME	**LEVEL**	**DISTANCE**	**HEART RATE**	**CALORIES**

NAME / TYPE:				
TIME	**LEVEL**	**DISTANCE**	**HEART RATE**	**CALORIES**

NOTES / OTHER

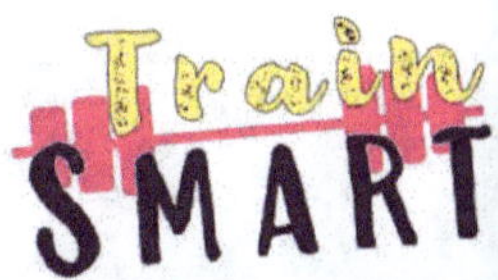

SESSION LOGBOOK

MON	TUE	WED	THU	FRI	SAT	SUN

Date:	Start Time:	Finish Time:

Session Name / Type:

STRENGTH & CONDITIONING

EXERCISE	SET 1	SET 2	SET 3	SET 4	SET 5
	REPS LOAD	REPS LOAD	REPS LOAD	REPS LOAD	REPS LOAD
	REPS LOAD	REPS LOAD	REPS LOAD	REPS LOAD	REPS LOAD
	REPS LOAD	REPS LOAD	REPS LOAD	REPS LOAD	REPS LOAD
	REPS LOAD	REPS LOAD	REPS LOAD	REPS LOAD	REPS LOAD
	REPS LOAD	REPS LOAD	REPS LOAD	REPS LOAD	REPS LOAD
	REPS LOAD	REPS LOAD	REPS LOAD	REPS LOAD	REPS LOAD
	REPS LOAD	REPS LOAD	REPS LOAD	REPS LOAD	REPS LOAD
	REPS LOAD	REPS LOAD	REPS LOAD	REPS LOAD	REPS LOAD
	REPS LOAD	REPS LOAD	REPS LOAD	REPS LOAD	REPS LOAD
	REPS LOAD	REPS LOAD	REPS LOAD	REPS LOAD	REPS LOAD

CARDIO

NAME / TYPE:				
TIME	**LEVEL**	**DISTANCE**	**HEART RATE**	**CALORIES**

NAME / TYPE:				
TIME	**LEVEL**	**DISTANCE**	**HEART RATE**	**CALORIES**

NOTES / OTHER

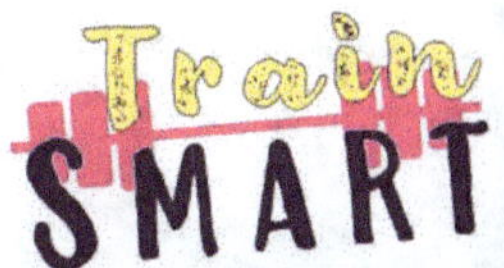

SESSION LOGBOOK

MON	TUE	WED	THU	FRI	SAT	SUN

Date:	Start Time:	Finish Time:

Session Name / Type:

STRENGTH & CONDITIONING

EXERCISE	SET 1	SET 2	SET 3	SET 4	SET 5
	REPS	REPS	REPS	REPS	REPS
	LOAD	LOAD	LOAD	LOAD	LOAD
	REPS	REPS	REPS	REPS	REPS
	LOAD	LOAD	LOAD	LOAD	LOAD
	REPS	REPS	REPS	REPS	REPS
	LOAD	LOAD	LOAD	LOAD	LOAD
	REPS	REPS	REPS	REPS	REPS
	LOAD	LOAD	LOAD	LOAD	LOAD
	REPS	REPS	REPS	REPS	REPS
	LOAD	LOAD	LOAD	LOAD	LOAD
	REPS	REPS	REPS	REPS	REPS
	LOAD	LOAD	LOAD	LOAD	LOAD
	REPS	REPS	REPS	REPS	REPS
	LOAD	LOAD	LOAD	LOAD	LOAD
	REPS	REPS	REPS	REPS	REPS
	LOAD	LOAD	LOAD	LOAD	LOAD
	REPS	REPS	REPS	REPS	REPS
	LOAD	LOAD	LOAD	LOAD	LOAD
	REPS	REPS	REPS	REPS	REPS
	LOAD	LOAD	LOAD	LOAD	LOAD

CARDIO

NAME / TYPE:				
TIME	**LEVEL**	**DISTANCE**	**HEART RATE**	**CALORIES**

NAME / TYPE:				
TIME	**LEVEL**	**DISTANCE**	**HEART RATE**	**CALORIES**

NOTES / OTHER

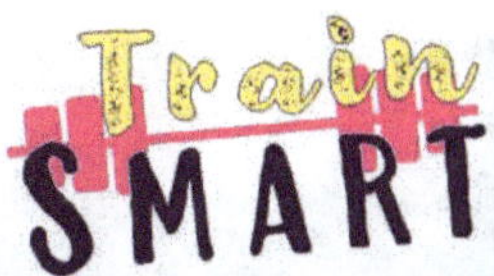

SESSION LOGBOOK

MON	TUE	WED	THU	FRI	SAT	SUN

Date:	Start Time:	Finish Time:

Session Name / Type:

STRENGTH & CONDITIONING

EXERCISE	SET 1	SET 2	SET 3	SET 4	SET 5
	REPS	REPS	REPS	REPS	REPS
	LOAD	LOAD	LOAD	LOAD	LOAD
	REPS	REPS	REPS	REPS	REPS
	LOAD	LOAD	LOAD	LOAD	LOAD
	REPS	REPS	REPS	REPS	REPS
	LOAD	LOAD	LOAD	LOAD	LOAD
	REPS	REPS	REPS	REPS	REPS
	LOAD	LOAD	LOAD	LOAD	LOAD
	REPS	REPS	REPS	REPS	REPS
	LOAD	LOAD	LOAD	LOAD	LOAD
	REPS	REPS	REPS	REPS	REPS
	LOAD	LOAD	LOAD	LOAD	LOAD
	REPS	REPS	REPS	REPS	REPS
	LOAD	LOAD	LOAD	LOAD	LOAD
	REPS	REPS	REPS	REPS	REPS
	LOAD	LOAD	LOAD	LOAD	LOAD
	REPS	REPS	REPS	REPS	REPS
	LOAD	LOAD	LOAD	LOAD	LOAD
	REPS	REPS	REPS	REPS	REPS
	LOAD	LOAD	LOAD	LOAD	LOAD

CARDIO

NAME / TYPE:				
TIME	**LEVEL**	**DISTANCE**	**HEART RATE**	**CALORIES**

NAME / TYPE:				
TIME	**LEVEL**	**DISTANCE**	**HEART RATE**	**CALORIES**

NOTES / OTHER

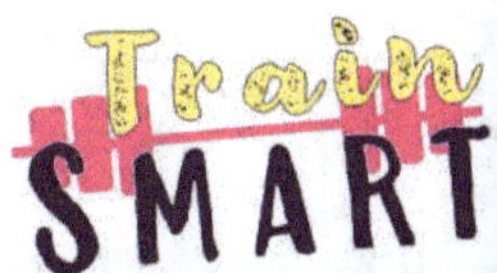

SESSION LOGBOOK

MON	TUE	WED	THU	FRI	SAT	SUN

Date:	Start Time:	Finish Time:

Session Name / Type:

STRENGTH & CONDITIONING

EXERCISE	SET 1	SET 2	SET 3	SET 4	SET 5
	REPS	REPS	REPS	REPS	REPS
	LOAD	LOAD	LOAD	LOAD	LOAD
	REPS	REPS	REPS	REPS	REPS
	LOAD	LOAD	LOAD	LOAD	LOAD
	REPS	REPS	REPS	REPS	REPS
	LOAD	LOAD	LOAD	LOAD	LOAD
	REPS	REPS	REPS	REPS	REPS
	LOAD	LOAD	LOAD	LOAD	LOAD
	REPS	REPS	REPS	REPS	REPS
	LOAD	LOAD	LOAD	LOAD	LOAD
	REPS	REPS	REPS	REPS	REPS
	LOAD	LOAD	LOAD	LOAD	LOAD
	REPS	REPS	REPS	REPS	REPS
	LOAD	LOAD	LOAD	LOAD	LOAD
	REPS	REPS	REPS	REPS	REPS
	LOAD	LOAD	LOAD	LOAD	LOAD
	REPS	REPS	REPS	REPS	REPS
	LOAD	LOAD	LOAD	LOAD	LOAD
	REPS	REPS	REPS	REPS	REPS
	LOAD	LOAD	LOAD	LOAD	LOAD

CARDIO

NAME / TYPE:				
TIME	**LEVEL**	**DISTANCE**	**HEART RATE**	**CALORIES**

NAME / TYPE:				
TIME	**LEVEL**	**DISTANCE**	**HEART RATE**	**CALORIES**

NOTES / OTHER

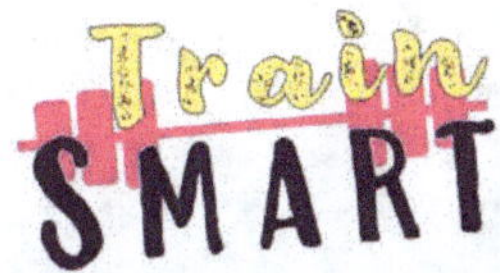

SESSION LOGBOOK

MON	TUE	WED	THU	FRI	SAT	SUN

Date:	Start Time:	Finish Time:

Session Name / Type:

STRENGTH & CONDITIONING

EXERCISE	SET 1	SET 2	SET 3	SET 4	SET 5
	REPS	REPS	REPS	REPS	REPS
	LOAD	LOAD	LOAD	LOAD	LOAD
	REPS	REPS	REPS	REPS	REPS
	LOAD	LOAD	LOAD	LOAD	LOAD
	REPS	REPS	REPS	REPS	REPS
	LOAD	LOAD	LOAD	LOAD	LOAD
	REPS	REPS	REPS	REPS	REPS
	LOAD	LOAD	LOAD	LOAD	LOAD
	REPS	REPS	REPS	REPS	REPS
	LOAD	LOAD	LOAD	LOAD	LOAD
	REPS	REPS	REPS	REPS	REPS
	LOAD	LOAD	LOAD	LOAD	LOAD
	REPS	REPS	REPS	REPS	REPS
	LOAD	LOAD	LOAD	LOAD	LOAD
	REPS	REPS	REPS	REPS	REPS
	LOAD	LOAD	LOAD	LOAD	LOAD
	REPS	REPS	REPS	REPS	REPS
	LOAD	LOAD	LOAD	LOAD	LOAD
	REPS	REPS	REPS	REPS	REPS
	LOAD	LOAD	LOAD	LOAD	LOAD

CARDIO

NAME / TYPE:				
TIME	**LEVEL**	**DISTANCE**	**HEART RATE**	**CALORIES**

NAME / TYPE:				
TIME	**LEVEL**	**DISTANCE**	**HEART RATE**	**CALORIES**

NOTES / OTHER

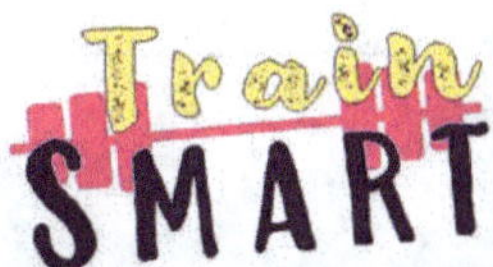

SESSION LOGBOOK

MON	TUE	WED	THU	FRI	SAT	SUN

Date:		Start Time:		Finish Time:	

Session Name / Type:

STRENGTH & CONDITIONING

EXERCISE	SET 1	SET 2	SET 3	SET 4	SET 5
	REPS	REPS	REPS	REPS	REPS
	LOAD	LOAD	LOAD	LOAD	LOAD
	REPS	REPS	REPS	REPS	REPS
	LOAD	LOAD	LOAD	LOAD	LOAD
	REPS	REPS	REPS	REPS	REPS
	LOAD	LOAD	LOAD	LOAD	LOAD
	REPS	REPS	REPS	REPS	REPS
	LOAD	LOAD	LOAD	LOAD	LOAD
	REPS	REPS	REPS	REPS	REPS
	LOAD	LOAD	LOAD	LOAD	LOAD
	REPS	REPS	REPS	REPS	REPS
	LOAD	LOAD	LOAD	LOAD	LOAD
	REPS	REPS	REPS	REPS	REPS
	LOAD	LOAD	LOAD	LOAD	LOAD
	REPS	REPS	REPS	REPS	REPS
	LOAD	LOAD	LOAD	LOAD	LOAD
	REPS	REPS	REPS	REPS	REPS
	LOAD	LOAD	LOAD	LOAD	LOAD
	REPS	REPS	REPS	REPS	REPS
	LOAD	LOAD	LOAD	LOAD	LOAD

CARDIO

NAME / TYPE:				
TIME	**LEVEL**	**DISTANCE**	**HEART RATE**	**CALORIES**

NAME / TYPE:				
TIME	**LEVEL**	**DISTANCE**	**HEART RATE**	**CALORIES**

NOTES / OTHER

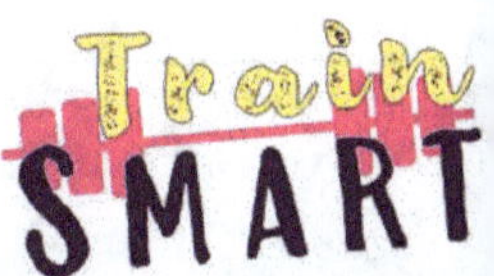

SESSION LOGBOOK

MON	TUE	WED	THU	FRI	SAT	SUN

Date:	Start Time:	Finish Time:

Session Name / Type:

STRENGTH & CONDITIONING

EXERCISE	SET 1	SET 2	SET 3	SET 4	SET 5
	REPS	REPS	REPS	REPS	REPS
	LOAD	LOAD	LOAD	LOAD	LOAD
	REPS	REPS	REPS	REPS	REPS
	LOAD	LOAD	LOAD	LOAD	LOAD
	REPS	REPS	REPS	REPS	REPS
	LOAD	LOAD	LOAD	LOAD	LOAD
	REPS	REPS	REPS	REPS	REPS
	LOAD	LOAD	LOAD	LOAD	LOAD
	REPS	REPS	REPS	REPS	REPS
	LOAD	LOAD	LOAD	LOAD	LOAD
	REPS	REPS	REPS	REPS	REPS
	LOAD	LOAD	LOAD	LOAD	LOAD
	REPS	REPS	REPS	REPS	REPS
	LOAD	LOAD	LOAD	LOAD	LOAD
	REPS	REPS	REPS	REPS	REPS
	LOAD	LOAD	LOAD	LOAD	LOAD
	REPS	REPS	REPS	REPS	REPS
	LOAD	LOAD	LOAD	LOAD	LOAD
	REPS	REPS	REPS	REPS	REPS
	LOAD	LOAD	LOAD	LOAD	LOAD

CARDIO

NAME / TYPE:				
TIME	**LEVEL**	**DISTANCE**	**HEART RATE**	**CALORIES**

NAME / TYPE:				
TIME	**LEVEL**	**DISTANCE**	**HEART RATE**	**CALORIES**

NOTES / OTHER

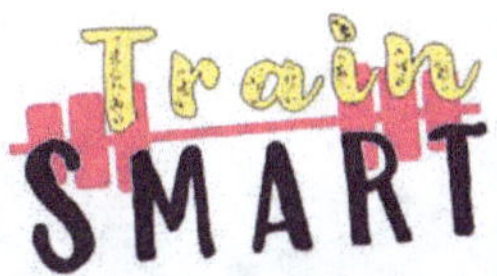

SESSION LOGBOOK

MON	TUE	WED	THU	FRI	SAT	SUN

Date:	Start Time:	Finish Time:

Session Name / Type:

STRENGTH & CONDITIONING

EXERCISE	SET 1	SET 2	SET 3	SET 4	SET 5
	REPS	REPS	REPS	REPS	REPS
	LOAD	LOAD	LOAD	LOAD	LOAD
	REPS	REPS	REPS	REPS	REPS
	LOAD	LOAD	LOAD	LOAD	LOAD
	REPS	REPS	REPS	REPS	REPS
	LOAD	LOAD	LOAD	LOAD	LOAD
	REPS	REPS	REPS	REPS	REPS
	LOAD	LOAD	LOAD	LOAD	LOAD
	REPS	REPS	REPS	REPS	REPS
	LOAD	LOAD	LOAD	LOAD	LOAD
	REPS	REPS	REPS	REPS	REPS
	LOAD	LOAD	LOAD	LOAD	LOAD
	REPS	REPS	REPS	REPS	REPS
	LOAD	LOAD	LOAD	LOAD	LOAD
	REPS	REPS	REPS	REPS	REPS
	LOAD	LOAD	LOAD	LOAD	LOAD
	REPS	REPS	REPS	REPS	REPS
	LOAD	LOAD	LOAD	LOAD	LOAD
	REPS	REPS	REPS	REPS	REPS
	LOAD	LOAD	LOAD	LOAD	LOAD

CARDIO

NAME / TYPE:				
TIME	**LEVEL**	**DISTANCE**	**HEART RATE**	**CALORIES**

NAME / TYPE:				
TIME	**LEVEL**	**DISTANCE**	**HEART RATE**	**CALORIES**

NOTES / OTHER

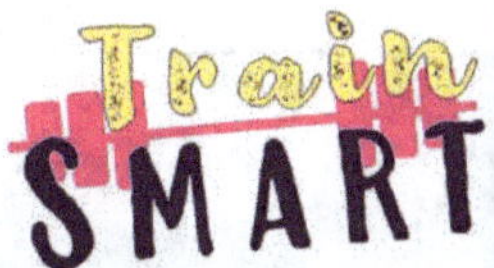

SESSION LOGBOOK

MON	TUE	WED	THU	FRI	SAT	SUN

Date:	Start Time:	Finish Time:

Session Name / Type:

STRENGTH & CONDITIONING

EXERCISE	SET 1	SET 2	SET 3	SET 4	SET 5
	REPS	REPS	REPS	REPS	REPS
	LOAD	LOAD	LOAD	LOAD	LOAD
	REPS	REPS	REPS	REPS	REPS
	LOAD	LOAD	LOAD	LOAD	LOAD
	REPS	REPS	REPS	REPS	REPS
	LOAD	LOAD	LOAD	LOAD	LOAD
	REPS	REPS	REPS	REPS	REPS
	LOAD	LOAD	LOAD	LOAD	LOAD
	REPS	REPS	REPS	REPS	REPS
	LOAD	LOAD	LOAD	LOAD	LOAD
	REPS	REPS	REPS	REPS	REPS
	LOAD	LOAD	LOAD	LOAD	LOAD
	REPS	REPS	REPS	REPS	REPS
	LOAD	LOAD	LOAD	LOAD	LOAD
	REPS	REPS	REPS	REPS	REPS
	LOAD	LOAD	LOAD	LOAD	LOAD
	REPS	REPS	REPS	REPS	REPS
	LOAD	LOAD	LOAD	LOAD	LOAD
	REPS	REPS	REPS	REPS	REPS
	LOAD	LOAD	LOAD	LOAD	LOAD

CARDIO

NAME / TYPE:				
TIME	**LEVEL**	**DISTANCE**	**HEART RATE**	**CALORIES**

NAME / TYPE:				
TIME	**LEVEL**	**DISTANCE**	**HEART RATE**	**CALORIES**

NOTES / OTHER

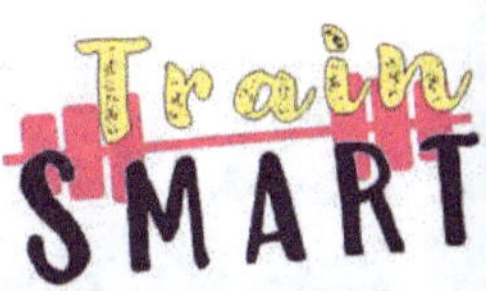

SESSION LOGBOOK

MON	TUE	WED	THU	FRI	SAT	SUN

Date:	Start Time:	Finish Time:

Session Name / Type:

STRENGTH & CONDITIONING

EXERCISE	SET 1	SET 2	SET 3	SET 4	SET 5
	REPS LOAD	REPS LOAD	REPS LOAD	REPS LOAD	REPS LOAD
	REPS LOAD	REPS LOAD	REPS LOAD	REPS LOAD	REPS LOAD
	REPS LOAD	REPS LOAD	REPS LOAD	REPS LOAD	REPS LOAD
	REPS LOAD	REPS LOAD	REPS LOAD	REPS LOAD	REPS LOAD
	REPS LOAD	REPS LOAD	REPS LOAD	REPS LOAD	REPS LOAD
	REPS LOAD	REPS LOAD	REPS LOAD	REPS LOAD	REPS LOAD
	REPS LOAD	REPS LOAD	REPS LOAD	REPS LOAD	REPS LOAD
	REPS LOAD	REPS LOAD	REPS LOAD	REPS LOAD	REPS LOAD
	REPS LOAD	REPS LOAD	REPS LOAD	REPS LOAD	REPS LOAD
	REPS LOAD	REPS LOAD	REPS LOAD	REPS LOAD	REPS LOAD

CARDIO

NAME / TYPE:				
TIME	**LEVEL**	**DISTANCE**	**HEART RATE**	**CALORIES**

NAME / TYPE:				
TIME	**LEVEL**	**DISTANCE**	**HEART RATE**	**CALORIES**

NOTES / OTHER

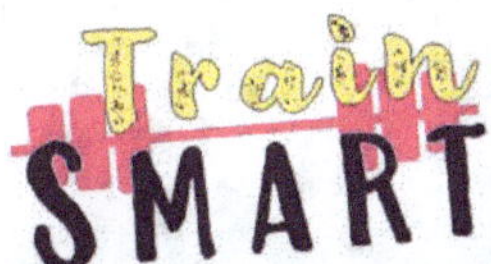

SESSION LOGBOOK

MON	TUE	WED	THU	FRI	SAT	SUN

Date:	Start Time:	Finish Time:

Session Name / Type:

STRENGTH & CONDITIONING

EXERCISE	SET 1	SET 2	SET 3	SET 4	SET 5
	REPS	REPS	REPS	REPS	REPS
	LOAD	LOAD	LOAD	LOAD	LOAD
	REPS	REPS	REPS	REPS	REPS
	LOAD	LOAD	LOAD	LOAD	LOAD
	REPS	REPS	REPS	REPS	REPS
	LOAD	LOAD	LOAD	LOAD	LOAD
	REPS	REPS	REPS	REPS	REPS
	LOAD	LOAD	LOAD	LOAD	LOAD
	REPS	REPS	REPS	REPS	REPS
	LOAD	LOAD	LOAD	LOAD	LOAD
	REPS	REPS	REPS	REPS	REPS
	LOAD	LOAD	LOAD	LOAD	LOAD
	REPS	REPS	REPS	REPS	REPS
	LOAD	LOAD	LOAD	LOAD	LOAD
	REPS	REPS	REPS	REPS	REPS
	LOAD	LOAD	LOAD	LOAD	LOAD
	REPS	REPS	REPS	REPS	REPS
	LOAD	LOAD	LOAD	LOAD	LOAD
	REPS	REPS	REPS	REPS	REPS
	LOAD	LOAD	LOAD	LOAD	LOAD

CARDIO

NAME / TYPE:				
TIME	**LEVEL**	**DISTANCE**	**HEART RATE**	**CALORIES**

NAME / TYPE:				
TIME	**LEVEL**	**DISTANCE**	**HEART RATE**	**CALORIES**

NOTES / OTHER

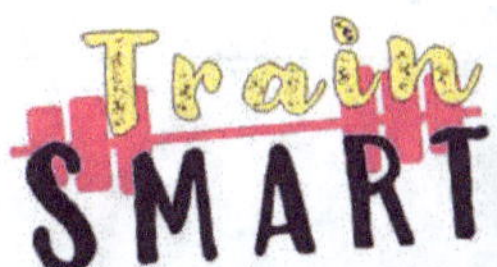

SESSION LOGBOOK

MON	TUE	WED	THU	FRI	SAT	SUN

Date:	Start Time:	Finish Time:

Session Name / Type:

STRENGTH & CONDITIONING

EXERCISE	SET 1	SET 2	SET 3	SET 4	SET 5
	REPS	REPS	REPS	REPS	REPS
	LOAD	LOAD	LOAD	LOAD	LOAD
	REPS	REPS	REPS	REPS	REPS
	LOAD	LOAD	LOAD	LOAD	LOAD
	REPS	REPS	REPS	REPS	REPS
	LOAD	LOAD	LOAD	LOAD	LOAD
	REPS	REPS	REPS	REPS	REPS
	LOAD	LOAD	LOAD	LOAD	LOAD
	REPS	REPS	REPS	REPS	REPS
	LOAD	LOAD	LOAD	LOAD	LOAD
	REPS	REPS	REPS	REPS	REPS
	LOAD	LOAD	LOAD	LOAD	LOAD
	REPS	REPS	REPS	REPS	REPS
	LOAD	LOAD	LOAD	LOAD	LOAD
	REPS	REPS	REPS	REPS	REPS
	LOAD	LOAD	LOAD	LOAD	LOAD
	REPS	REPS	REPS	REPS	REPS
	LOAD	LOAD	LOAD	LOAD	LOAD
	REPS	REPS	REPS	REPS	REPS
	LOAD	LOAD	LOAD	LOAD	LOAD

CARDIO

NAME / TYPE:				
TIME	**LEVEL**	**DISTANCE**	**HEART RATE**	**CALORIES**

NAME / TYPE:				
TIME	**LEVEL**	**DISTANCE**	**HEART RATE**	**CALORIES**

NOTES / OTHER

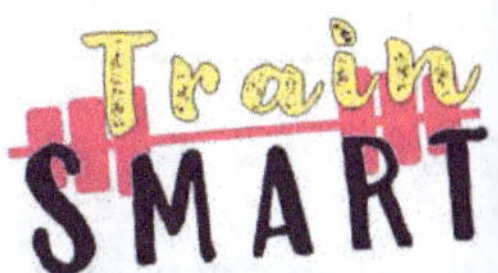

SESSION LOGBOOK

MON	TUE	WED	THU	FRI	SAT	SUN

Date:	Start Time:	Finish Time:

Session Name / Type:

STRENGTH & CONDITIONING

EXERCISE	SET 1	SET 2	SET 3	SET 4	SET 5
	REPS	REPS	REPS	REPS	REPS
	LOAD	LOAD	LOAD	LOAD	LOAD
	REPS	REPS	REPS	REPS	REPS
	LOAD	LOAD	LOAD	LOAD	LOAD
	REPS	REPS	REPS	REPS	REPS
	LOAD	LOAD	LOAD	LOAD	LOAD
	REPS	REPS	REPS	REPS	REPS
	LOAD	LOAD	LOAD	LOAD	LOAD
	REPS	REPS	REPS	REPS	REPS
	LOAD	LOAD	LOAD	LOAD	LOAD
	REPS	REPS	REPS	REPS	REPS
	LOAD	LOAD	LOAD	LOAD	LOAD
	REPS	REPS	REPS	REPS	REPS
	LOAD	LOAD	LOAD	LOAD	LOAD
	REPS	REPS	REPS	REPS	REPS
	LOAD	LOAD	LOAD	LOAD	LOAD
	REPS	REPS	REPS	REPS	REPS
	LOAD	LOAD	LOAD	LOAD	LOAD
	REPS	REPS	REPS	REPS	REPS
	LOAD	LOAD	LOAD	LOAD	LOAD

CARDIO

NAME / TYPE:				
TIME	**LEVEL**	**DISTANCE**	**HEART RATE**	**CALORIES**

NAME / TYPE:				
TIME	**LEVEL**	**DISTANCE**	**HEART RATE**	**CALORIES**

NOTES / OTHER

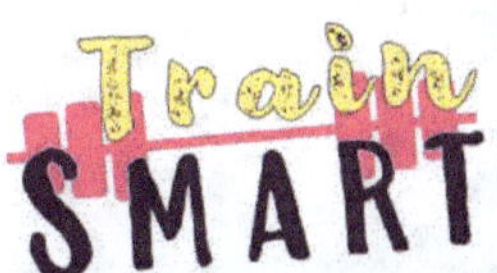

SESSION LOGBOOK

MON	TUE	WED	THU	FRI	SAT	SUN

Date:	Start Time:	Finish Time:

Session Name / Type:

STRENGTH & CONDITIONING

EXERCISE	SET 1	SET 2	SET 3	SET 4	SET 5
	REPS	REPS	REPS	REPS	REPS
	LOAD	LOAD	LOAD	LOAD	LOAD
	REPS	REPS	REPS	REPS	REPS
	LOAD	LOAD	LOAD	LOAD	LOAD
	REPS	REPS	REPS	REPS	REPS
	LOAD	LOAD	LOAD	LOAD	LOAD
	REPS	REPS	REPS	REPS	REPS
	LOAD	LOAD	LOAD	LOAD	LOAD
	REPS	REPS	REPS	REPS	REPS
	LOAD	LOAD	LOAD	LOAD	LOAD
	REPS	REPS	REPS	REPS	REPS
	LOAD	LOAD	LOAD	LOAD	LOAD
	REPS	REPS	REPS	REPS	REPS
	LOAD	LOAD	LOAD	LOAD	LOAD
	REPS	REPS	REPS	REPS	REPS
	LOAD	LOAD	LOAD	LOAD	LOAD
	REPS	REPS	REPS	REPS	REPS
	LOAD	LOAD	LOAD	LOAD	LOAD
	REPS	REPS	REPS	REPS	REPS
	LOAD	LOAD	LOAD	LOAD	LOAD

CARDIO

NAME / TYPE:				
TIME	**LEVEL**	**DISTANCE**	**HEART RATE**	**CALORIES**

NAME / TYPE:				
TIME	**LEVEL**	**DISTANCE**	**HEART RATE**	**CALORIES**

NOTES / OTHER

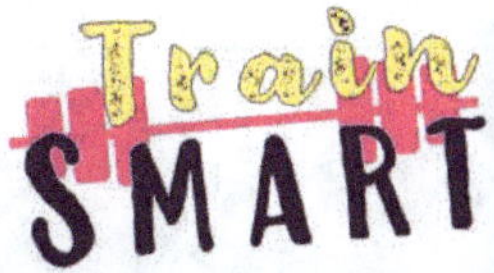

SESSION LOGBOOK

MON	TUE	WED	THU	FRI	SAT	SUN

Date:	Start Time:	Finish Time:

Session Name / Type:

STRENGTH & CONDITIONING

EXERCISE	SET 1	SET 2	SET 3	SET 4	SET 5
	REPS LOAD	REPS LOAD	REPS LOAD	REPS LOAD	REPS LOAD
	REPS LOAD	REPS LOAD	REPS LOAD	REPS LOAD	REPS LOAD
	REPS LOAD	REPS LOAD	REPS LOAD	REPS LOAD	REPS LOAD
	REPS LOAD	REPS LOAD	REPS LOAD	REPS LOAD	REPS LOAD
	REPS LOAD	REPS LOAD	REPS LOAD	REPS LOAD	REPS LOAD
	REPS LOAD	REPS LOAD	REPS LOAD	REPS LOAD	REPS LOAD
	REPS LOAD	REPS LOAD	REPS LOAD	REPS LOAD	REPS LOAD
	REPS LOAD	REPS LOAD	REPS LOAD	REPS LOAD	REPS LOAD
	REPS LOAD	REPS LOAD	REPS LOAD	REPS LOAD	REPS LOAD
	REPS LOAD	REPS LOAD	REPS LOAD	REPS LOAD	REPS LOAD

CARDIO

NAME / TYPE:				
TIME	**LEVEL**	**DISTANCE**	**HEART RATE**	**CALORIES**

NAME / TYPE:				
TIME	**LEVEL**	**DISTANCE**	**HEART RATE**	**CALORIES**

NOTES / OTHER

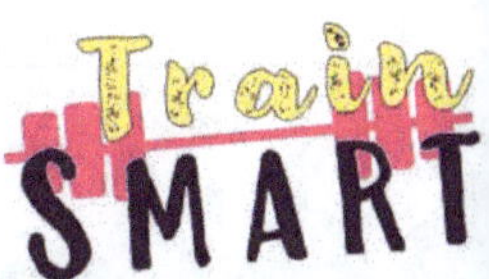

SESSION LOGBOOK

MON	TUE	WED	THU	FRI	SAT	SUN

Date:	Start Time:	Finish Time:

Session Name / Type:

STRENGTH & CONDITIONING

EXERCISE	SET 1	SET 2	SET 3	SET 4	SET 5
	REPS	REPS	REPS	REPS	REPS
	LOAD	LOAD	LOAD	LOAD	LOAD
	REPS	REPS	REPS	REPS	REPS
	LOAD	LOAD	LOAD	LOAD	LOAD
	REPS	REPS	REPS	REPS	REPS
	LOAD	LOAD	LOAD	LOAD	LOAD
	REPS	REPS	REPS	REPS	REPS
	LOAD	LOAD	LOAD	LOAD	LOAD
	REPS	REPS	REPS	REPS	REPS
	LOAD	LOAD	LOAD	LOAD	LOAD
	REPS	REPS	REPS	REPS	REPS
	LOAD	LOAD	LOAD	LOAD	LOAD
	REPS	REPS	REPS	REPS	REPS
	LOAD	LOAD	LOAD	LOAD	LOAD
	REPS	REPS	REPS	REPS	REPS
	LOAD	LOAD	LOAD	LOAD	LOAD
	REPS	REPS	REPS	REPS	REPS
	LOAD	LOAD	LOAD	LOAD	LOAD
	REPS	REPS	REPS	REPS	REPS
	LOAD	LOAD	LOAD	LOAD	LOAD

CARDIO

NAME / TYPE:				
TIME	LEVEL	DISTANCE	HEART RATE	CALORIES

NAME / TYPE:				
TIME	LEVEL	DISTANCE	HEART RATE	CALORIES

NOTES / OTHER

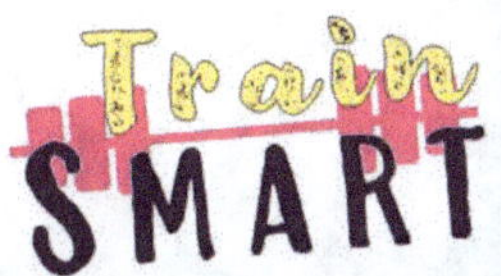

SESSION LOGBOOK

MON	TUE	WED	THU	FRI	SAT	SUN

Date:	Start Time:	Finish Time:

Session Name / Type:

STRENGTH & CONDITIONING

EXERCISE	SET 1	SET 2	SET 3	SET 4	SET 5
	REPS	REPS	REPS	REPS	REPS
	LOAD	LOAD	LOAD	LOAD	LOAD
	REPS	REPS	REPS	REPS	REPS
	LOAD	LOAD	LOAD	LOAD	LOAD
	REPS	REPS	REPS	REPS	REPS
	LOAD	LOAD	LOAD	LOAD	LOAD
	REPS	REPS	REPS	REPS	REPS
	LOAD	LOAD	LOAD	LOAD	LOAD
	REPS	REPS	REPS	REPS	REPS
	LOAD	LOAD	LOAD	LOAD	LOAD
	REPS	REPS	REPS	REPS	REPS
	LOAD	LOAD	LOAD	LOAD	LOAD
	REPS	REPS	REPS	REPS	REPS
	LOAD	LOAD	LOAD	LOAD	LOAD
	REPS	REPS	REPS	REPS	REPS
	LOAD	LOAD	LOAD	LOAD	LOAD
	REPS	REPS	REPS	REPS	REPS
	LOAD	LOAD	LOAD	LOAD	LOAD
	REPS	REPS	REPS	REPS	REPS
	LOAD	LOAD	LOAD	LOAD	LOAD

CARDIO

NAME / TYPE:				
TIME	**LEVEL**	**DISTANCE**	**HEART RATE**	**CALORIES**

NAME / TYPE:				
TIME	**LEVEL**	**DISTANCE**	**HEART RATE**	**CALORIES**

NOTES / OTHER

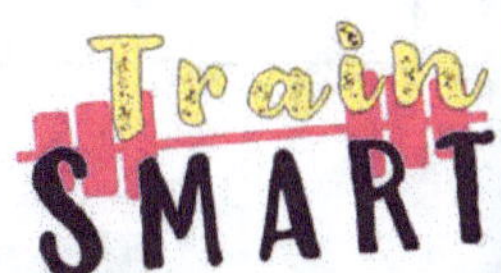

SESSION LOGBOOK

MON	TUE	WED	THU	FRI	SAT	SUN

Date:	Start Time:	Finish Time:

Session Name / Type:

STRENGTH & CONDITIONING

EXERCISE	SET 1	SET 2	SET 3	SET 4	SET 5
	REPS	REPS	REPS	REPS	REPS
	LOAD	LOAD	LOAD	LOAD	LOAD
	REPS	REPS	REPS	REPS	REPS
	LOAD	LOAD	LOAD	LOAD	LOAD
	REPS	REPS	REPS	REPS	REPS
	LOAD	LOAD	LOAD	LOAD	LOAD
	REPS	REPS	REPS	REPS	REPS
	LOAD	LOAD	LOAD	LOAD	LOAD
	REPS	REPS	REPS	REPS	REPS
	LOAD	LOAD	LOAD	LOAD	LOAD
	REPS	REPS	REPS	REPS	REPS
	LOAD	LOAD	LOAD	LOAD	LOAD
	REPS	REPS	REPS	REPS	REPS
	LOAD	LOAD	LOAD	LOAD	LOAD
	REPS	REPS	REPS	REPS	REPS
	LOAD	LOAD	LOAD	LOAD	LOAD
	REPS	REPS	REPS	REPS	REPS
	LOAD	LOAD	LOAD	LOAD	LOAD
	REPS	REPS	REPS	REPS	REPS
	LOAD	LOAD	LOAD	LOAD	LOAD

CARDIO

NAME / TYPE:				
TIME	LEVEL	DISTANCE	HEART RATE	CALORIES

NAME / TYPE:				
TIME	LEVEL	DISTANCE	HEART RATE	CALORIES

NOTES / OTHER

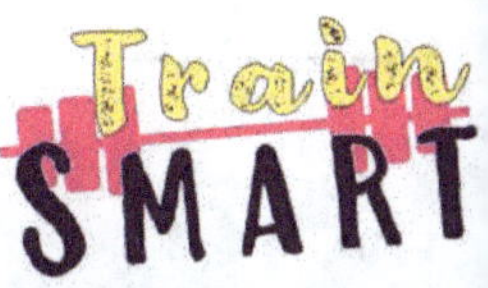

SESSION LOGBOOK

MON	TUE	WED	THU	FRI	SAT	SUN

Date:	Start Time:	Finish Time:

Session Name / Type:

STRENGTH & CONDITIONING

EXERCISE	SET 1	SET 2	SET 3	SET 4	SET 5
	REPS	REPS	REPS	REPS	REPS
	LOAD	LOAD	LOAD	LOAD	LOAD
	REPS	REPS	REPS	REPS	REPS
	LOAD	LOAD	LOAD	LOAD	LOAD
	REPS	REPS	REPS	REPS	REPS
	LOAD	LOAD	LOAD	LOAD	LOAD
	REPS	REPS	REPS	REPS	REPS
	LOAD	LOAD	LOAD	LOAD	LOAD
	REPS	REPS	REPS	REPS	REPS
	LOAD	LOAD	LOAD	LOAD	LOAD
	REPS	REPS	REPS	REPS	REPS
	LOAD	LOAD	LOAD	LOAD	LOAD
	REPS	REPS	REPS	REPS	REPS
	LOAD	LOAD	LOAD	LOAD	LOAD
	REPS	REPS	REPS	REPS	REPS
	LOAD	LOAD	LOAD	LOAD	LOAD
	REPS	REPS	REPS	REPS	REPS
	LOAD	LOAD	LOAD	LOAD	LOAD
	REPS	REPS	REPS	REPS	REPS
	LOAD	LOAD	LOAD	LOAD	LOAD

CARDIO

NAME / TYPE:				
TIME	**LEVEL**	**DISTANCE**	**HEART RATE**	**CALORIES**

NAME / TYPE:				
TIME	**LEVEL**	**DISTANCE**	**HEART RATE**	**CALORIES**

NOTES / OTHER

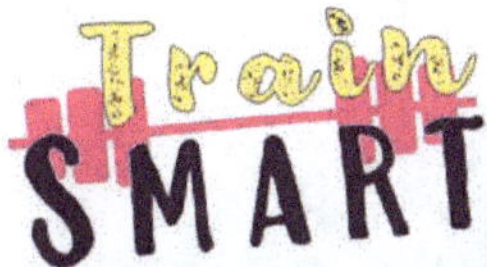

SESSION LOGBOOK

MON	TUE	WED	THU	FRI	SAT	SUN

Date:	Start Time:	Finish Time:

Session Name / Type:

STRENGTH & CONDITIONING

EXERCISE	SET 1	SET 2	SET 3	SET 4	SET 5
	REPS	REPS	REPS	REPS	REPS
	LOAD	LOAD	LOAD	LOAD	LOAD
	REPS	REPS	REPS	REPS	REPS
	LOAD	LOAD	LOAD	LOAD	LOAD
	REPS	REPS	REPS	REPS	REPS
	LOAD	LOAD	LOAD	LOAD	LOAD
	REPS	REPS	REPS	REPS	REPS
	LOAD	LOAD	LOAD	LOAD	LOAD
	REPS	REPS	REPS	REPS	REPS
	LOAD	LOAD	LOAD	LOAD	LOAD
	REPS	REPS	REPS	REPS	REPS
	LOAD	LOAD	LOAD	LOAD	LOAD
	REPS	REPS	REPS	REPS	REPS
	LOAD	LOAD	LOAD	LOAD	LOAD
	REPS	REPS	REPS	REPS	REPS
	LOAD	LOAD	LOAD	LOAD	LOAD
	REPS	REPS	REPS	REPS	REPS
	LOAD	LOAD	LOAD	LOAD	LOAD
	REPS	REPS	REPS	REPS	REPS
	LOAD	LOAD	LOAD	LOAD	LOAD

CARDIO

NAME / TYPE:				
TIME	LEVEL	DISTANCE	HEART RATE	CALORIES

NAME / TYPE:				
TIME	LEVEL	DISTANCE	HEART RATE	CALORIES

NOTES / OTHER

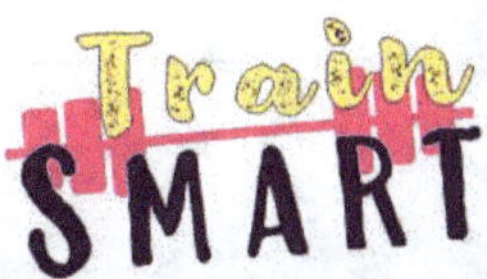

SESSION LOGBOOK

MON	TUE	WED	THU	FRI	SAT	SUN

Date:	Start Time:	Finish Time:

Session Name / Type:

STRENGTH & CONDITIONING

EXERCISE	SET 1	SET 2	SET 3	SET 4	SET 5
	REPS	REPS	REPS	REPS	REPS
	LOAD	LOAD	LOAD	LOAD	LOAD
	REPS	REPS	REPS	REPS	REPS
	LOAD	LOAD	LOAD	LOAD	LOAD
	REPS	REPS	REPS	REPS	REPS
	LOAD	LOAD	LOAD	LOAD	LOAD
	REPS	REPS	REPS	REPS	REPS
	LOAD	LOAD	LOAD	LOAD	LOAD
	REPS	REPS	REPS	REPS	REPS
	LOAD	LOAD	LOAD	LOAD	LOAD
	REPS	REPS	REPS	REPS	REPS
	LOAD	LOAD	LOAD	LOAD	LOAD
	REPS	REPS	REPS	REPS	REPS
	LOAD	LOAD	LOAD	LOAD	LOAD
	REPS	REPS	REPS	REPS	REPS
	LOAD	LOAD	LOAD	LOAD	LOAD
	REPS	REPS	REPS	REPS	REPS
	LOAD	LOAD	LOAD	LOAD	LOAD
	REPS	REPS	REPS	REPS	REPS
	LOAD	LOAD	LOAD	LOAD	LOAD

CARDIO

NAME / TYPE:				
TIME	LEVEL	DISTANCE	HEART RATE	CALORIES

NAME / TYPE:				
TIME	LEVEL	DISTANCE	HEART RATE	CALORIES

NOTES / OTHER

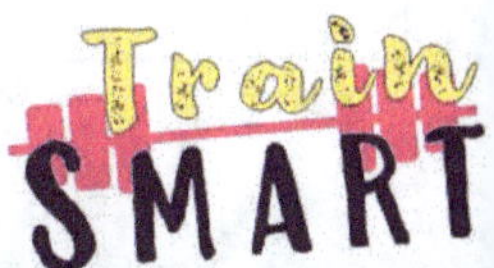

SESSION LOGBOOK

MON	TUE	WED	THU	FRI	SAT	SUN

Date:	Start Time:	Finish Time:

Session Name / Type:

STRENGTH & CONDITIONING

EXERCISE	SET 1	SET 2	SET 3	SET 4	SET 5
	REPS	REPS	REPS	REPS	REPS
	LOAD	LOAD	LOAD	LOAD	LOAD
	REPS	REPS	REPS	REPS	REPS
	LOAD	LOAD	LOAD	LOAD	LOAD
	REPS	REPS	REPS	REPS	REPS
	LOAD	LOAD	LOAD	LOAD	LOAD
	REPS	REPS	REPS	REPS	REPS
	LOAD	LOAD	LOAD	LOAD	LOAD
	REPS	REPS	REPS	REPS	REPS
	LOAD	LOAD	LOAD	LOAD	LOAD
	REPS	REPS	REPS	REPS	REPS
	LOAD	LOAD	LOAD	LOAD	LOAD
	REPS	REPS	REPS	REPS	REPS
	LOAD	LOAD	LOAD	LOAD	LOAD
	REPS	REPS	REPS	REPS	REPS
	LOAD	LOAD	LOAD	LOAD	LOAD
	REPS	REPS	REPS	REPS	REPS
	LOAD	LOAD	LOAD	LOAD	LOAD
	REPS	REPS	REPS	REPS	REPS
	LOAD	LOAD	LOAD	LOAD	LOAD

CARDIO

NAME / TYPE:				
TIME	**LEVEL**	**DISTANCE**	**HEART RATE**	**CALORIES**

NAME / TYPE:				
TIME	**LEVEL**	**DISTANCE**	**HEART RATE**	**CALORIES**

NOTES / OTHER

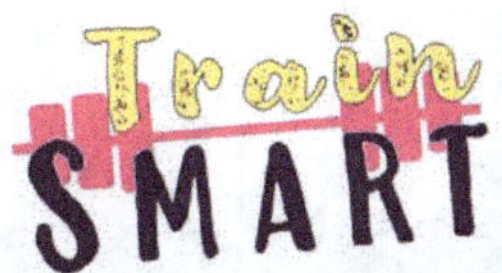

SESSION LOGBOOK

MON	TUE	WED	THU	FRI	SAT	SUN

Date:	Start Time:	Finish Time:

Session Name / Type:

STRENGTH & CONDITIONING

EXERCISE	SET 1	SET 2	SET 3	SET 4	SET 5
	REPS	REPS	REPS	REPS	REPS
	LOAD	LOAD	LOAD	LOAD	LOAD
	REPS	REPS	REPS	REPS	REPS
	LOAD	LOAD	LOAD	LOAD	LOAD
	REPS	REPS	REPS	REPS	REPS
	LOAD	LOAD	LOAD	LOAD	LOAD
	REPS	REPS	REPS	REPS	REPS
	LOAD	LOAD	LOAD	LOAD	LOAD
	REPS	REPS	REPS	REPS	REPS
	LOAD	LOAD	LOAD	LOAD	LOAD
	REPS	REPS	REPS	REPS	REPS
	LOAD	LOAD	LOAD	LOAD	LOAD
	REPS	REPS	REPS	REPS	REPS
	LOAD	LOAD	LOAD	LOAD	LOAD
	REPS	REPS	REPS	REPS	REPS
	LOAD	LOAD	LOAD	LOAD	LOAD
	REPS	REPS	REPS	REPS	REPS
	LOAD	LOAD	LOAD	LOAD	LOAD
	REPS	REPS	REPS	REPS	REPS
	LOAD	LOAD	LOAD	LOAD	LOAD

CARDIO

NAME / TYPE:				
TIME	**LEVEL**	**DISTANCE**	**HEART RATE**	**CALORIES**

NAME / TYPE:				
TIME	**LEVEL**	**DISTANCE**	**HEART RATE**	**CALORIES**

NOTES / OTHER

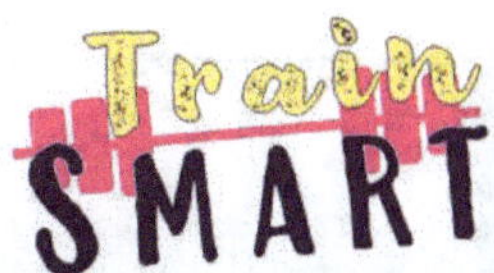

SESSION LOGBOOK

MON	TUE	WED	THU	FRI	SAT	SUN

Date:	Start Time:	Finish Time:

Session Name / Type:

STRENGTH & CONDITIONING

EXERCISE	SET 1	SET 2	SET 3	SET 4	SET 5
	REPS	REPS	REPS	REPS	REPS
	LOAD	LOAD	LOAD	LOAD	LOAD
	REPS	REPS	REPS	REPS	REPS
	LOAD	LOAD	LOAD	LOAD	LOAD
	REPS	REPS	REPS	REPS	REPS
	LOAD	LOAD	LOAD	LOAD	LOAD
	REPS	REPS	REPS	REPS	REPS
	LOAD	LOAD	LOAD	LOAD	LOAD
	REPS	REPS	REPS	REPS	REPS
	LOAD	LOAD	LOAD	LOAD	LOAD
	REPS	REPS	REPS	REPS	REPS
	LOAD	LOAD	LOAD	LOAD	LOAD
	REPS	REPS	REPS	REPS	REPS
	LOAD	LOAD	LOAD	LOAD	LOAD
	REPS	REPS	REPS	REPS	REPS
	LOAD	LOAD	LOAD	LOAD	LOAD
	REPS	REPS	REPS	REPS	REPS
	LOAD	LOAD	LOAD	LOAD	LOAD
	REPS	REPS	REPS	REPS	REPS
	LOAD	LOAD	LOAD	LOAD	LOAD

CARDIO

NAME / TYPE:				
TIME	**LEVEL**	**DISTANCE**	**HEART RATE**	**CALORIES**

NAME / TYPE:				
TIME	**LEVEL**	**DISTANCE**	**HEART RATE**	**CALORIES**

NOTES / OTHER

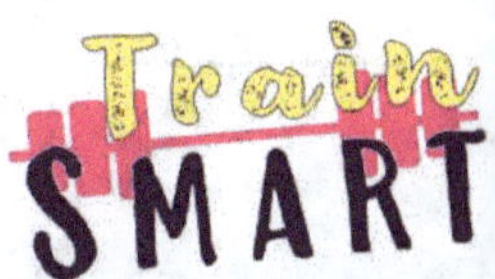

SESSION LOGBOOK

MON	TUE	WED	THU	FRI	SAT	SUN

Date:	Start Time:	Finish Time:

Session Name / Type:

STRENGTH & CONDITIONING

EXERCISE	SET 1	SET 2	SET 3	SET 4	SET 5
	REPS	REPS	REPS	REPS	REPS
	LOAD	LOAD	LOAD	LOAD	LOAD
	REPS	REPS	REPS	REPS	REPS
	LOAD	LOAD	LOAD	LOAD	LOAD
	REPS	REPS	REPS	REPS	REPS
	LOAD	LOAD	LOAD	LOAD	LOAD
	REPS	REPS	REPS	REPS	REPS
	LOAD	LOAD	LOAD	LOAD	LOAD
	REPS	REPS	REPS	REPS	REPS
	LOAD	LOAD	LOAD	LOAD	LOAD
	REPS	REPS	REPS	REPS	REPS
	LOAD	LOAD	LOAD	LOAD	LOAD
	REPS	REPS	REPS	REPS	REPS
	LOAD	LOAD	LOAD	LOAD	LOAD
	REPS	REPS	REPS	REPS	REPS
	LOAD	LOAD	LOAD	LOAD	LOAD
	REPS	REPS	REPS	REPS	REPS
	LOAD	LOAD	LOAD	LOAD	LOAD
	REPS	REPS	REPS	REPS	REPS
	LOAD	LOAD	LOAD	LOAD	LOAD

CARDIO

NAME / TYPE:				
TIME	**LEVEL**	**DISTANCE**	**HEART RATE**	**CALORIES**

NAME / TYPE:				
TIME	**LEVEL**	**DISTANCE**	**HEART RATE**	**CALORIES**

NOTES / OTHER

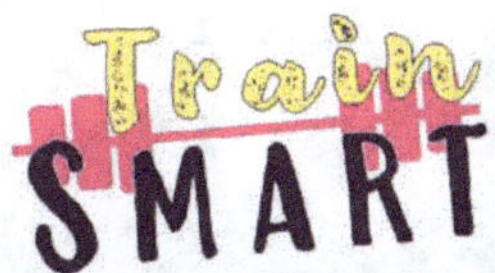

SESSION LOGBOOK

MON	TUE	WED	THU	FRI	SAT	SUN

Date:	Start Time:	Finish Time:

Session Name / Type:

STRENGTH & CONDITIONING

EXERCISE	SET 1	SET 2	SET 3	SET 4	SET 5
	REPS	REPS	REPS	REPS	REPS
	LOAD	LOAD	LOAD	LOAD	LOAD
	REPS	REPS	REPS	REPS	REPS
	LOAD	LOAD	LOAD	LOAD	LOAD
	REPS	REPS	REPS	REPS	REPS
	LOAD	LOAD	LOAD	LOAD	LOAD
	REPS	REPS	REPS	REPS	REPS
	LOAD	LOAD	LOAD	LOAD	LOAD
	REPS	REPS	REPS	REPS	REPS
	LOAD	LOAD	LOAD	LOAD	LOAD
	REPS	REPS	REPS	REPS	REPS
	LOAD	LOAD	LOAD	LOAD	LOAD
	REPS	REPS	REPS	REPS	REPS
	LOAD	LOAD	LOAD	LOAD	LOAD
	REPS	REPS	REPS	REPS	REPS
	LOAD	LOAD	LOAD	LOAD	LOAD
	REPS	REPS	REPS	REPS	REPS
	LOAD	LOAD	LOAD	LOAD	LOAD
	REPS	REPS	REPS	REPS	REPS
	LOAD	LOAD	LOAD	LOAD	LOAD

CARDIO

NAME / TYPE:				
TIME	**LEVEL**	**DISTANCE**	**HEART RATE**	**CALORIES**

NAME / TYPE:				
TIME	**LEVEL**	**DISTANCE**	**HEART RATE**	**CALORIES**

NOTES / OTHER

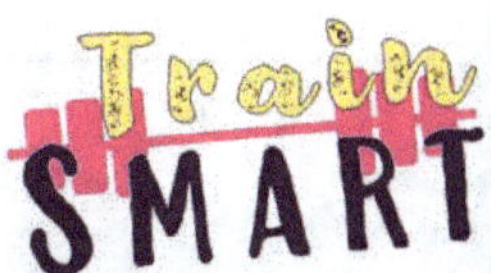

SESSION LOGBOOK

MON	TUE	WED	THU	FRI	SAT	SUN

Date:	Start Time:	Finish Time:

Session Name / Type:

STRENGTH & CONDITIONING

EXERCISE	SET 1	SET 2	SET 3	SET 4	SET 5
	REPS	REPS	REPS	REPS	REPS
	LOAD	LOAD	LOAD	LOAD	LOAD
	REPS	REPS	REPS	REPS	REPS
	LOAD	LOAD	LOAD	LOAD	LOAD
	REPS	REPS	REPS	REPS	REPS
	LOAD	LOAD	LOAD	LOAD	LOAD
	REPS	REPS	REPS	REPS	REPS
	LOAD	LOAD	LOAD	LOAD	LOAD
	REPS	REPS	REPS	REPS	REPS
	LOAD	LOAD	LOAD	LOAD	LOAD
	REPS	REPS	REPS	REPS	REPS
	LOAD	LOAD	LOAD	LOAD	LOAD
	REPS	REPS	REPS	REPS	REPS
	LOAD	LOAD	LOAD	LOAD	LOAD
	REPS	REPS	REPS	REPS	REPS
	LOAD	LOAD	LOAD	LOAD	LOAD
	REPS	REPS	REPS	REPS	REPS
	LOAD	LOAD	LOAD	LOAD	LOAD
	REPS	REPS	REPS	REPS	REPS
	LOAD	LOAD	LOAD	LOAD	LOAD

CARDIO

NAME / TYPE:				
TIME	**LEVEL**	**DISTANCE**	**HEART RATE**	**CALORIES**

NAME / TYPE:				
TIME	**LEVEL**	**DISTANCE**	**HEART RATE**	**CALORIES**

NOTES / OTHER

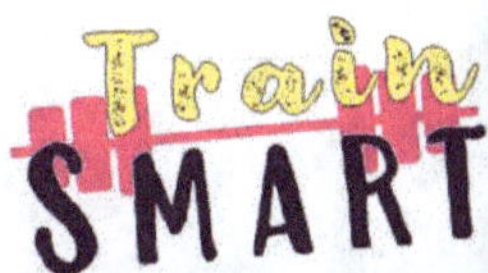

SESSION LOGBOOK

MON	TUE	WED	THU	FRI	SAT	SUN

Date:	Start Time:	Finish Time:

Session Name / Type:

STRENGTH & CONDITIONING

EXERCISE	SET 1	SET 2	SET 3	SET 4	SET 5
	REPS LOAD	REPS LOAD	REPS LOAD	REPS LOAD	REPS LOAD
	REPS LOAD	REPS LOAD	REPS LOAD	REPS LOAD	REPS LOAD
	REPS LOAD	REPS LOAD	REPS LOAD	REPS LOAD	REPS LOAD
	REPS LOAD	REPS LOAD	REPS LOAD	REPS LOAD	REPS LOAD
	REPS LOAD	REPS LOAD	REPS LOAD	REPS LOAD	REPS LOAD
	REPS LOAD	REPS LOAD	REPS LOAD	REPS LOAD	REPS LOAD
	REPS LOAD	REPS LOAD	REPS LOAD	REPS LOAD	REPS LOAD
	REPS LOAD	REPS LOAD	REPS LOAD	REPS LOAD	REPS LOAD
	REPS LOAD	REPS LOAD	REPS LOAD	REPS LOAD	REPS LOAD
	REPS LOAD	REPS LOAD	REPS LOAD	REPS LOAD	REPS LOAD

CARDIO

NAME / TYPE:				
TIME	LEVEL	DISTANCE	HEART RATE	CALORIES

NAME / TYPE:				
TIME	LEVEL	DISTANCE	HEART RATE	CALORIES

NOTES / OTHER

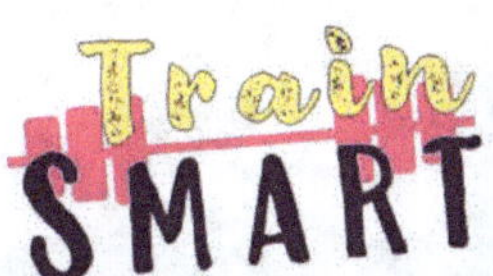

SESSION LOGBOOK

MON	TUE	WED	THU	FRI	SAT	SUN

Date:	Start Time:	Finish Time:

Session Name / Type:

STRENGTH & CONDITIONING

EXERCISE	SET 1	SET 2	SET 3	SET 4	SET 5
	REPS	REPS	REPS	REPS	REPS
	LOAD	LOAD	LOAD	LOAD	LOAD
	REPS	REPS	REPS	REPS	REPS
	LOAD	LOAD	LOAD	LOAD	LOAD
	REPS	REPS	REPS	REPS	REPS
	LOAD	LOAD	LOAD	LOAD	LOAD
	REPS	REPS	REPS	REPS	REPS
	LOAD	LOAD	LOAD	LOAD	LOAD
	REPS	REPS	REPS	REPS	REPS
	LOAD	LOAD	LOAD	LOAD	LOAD
	REPS	REPS	REPS	REPS	REPS
	LOAD	LOAD	LOAD	LOAD	LOAD
	REPS	REPS	REPS	REPS	REPS
	LOAD	LOAD	LOAD	LOAD	LOAD
	REPS	REPS	REPS	REPS	REPS
	LOAD	LOAD	LOAD	LOAD	LOAD
	REPS	REPS	REPS	REPS	REPS
	LOAD	LOAD	LOAD	LOAD	LOAD
	REPS	REPS	REPS	REPS	REPS
	LOAD	LOAD	LOAD	LOAD	LOAD

CARDIO

NAME / TYPE:				
TIME	**LEVEL**	**DISTANCE**	**HEART RATE**	**CALORIES**

NAME / TYPE:				
TIME	**LEVEL**	**DISTANCE**	**HEART RATE**	**CALORIES**

NOTES / OTHER

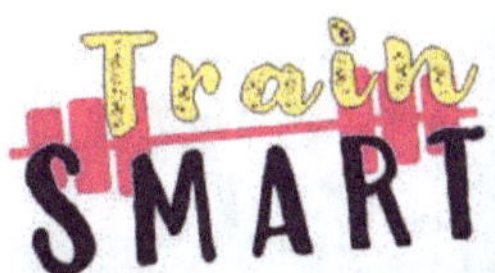

SESSION LOGBOOK

MON	TUE	WED	THU	FRI	SAT	SUN

Date:	Start Time:	Finish Time:

Session Name / Type:

STRENGTH & CONDITIONING

EXERCISE	SET 1	SET 2	SET 3	SET 4	SET 5
	REPS	REPS	REPS	REPS	REPS
	LOAD	LOAD	LOAD	LOAD	LOAD
	REPS	REPS	REPS	REPS	REPS
	LOAD	LOAD	LOAD	LOAD	LOAD
	REPS	REPS	REPS	REPS	REPS
	LOAD	LOAD	LOAD	LOAD	LOAD
	REPS	REPS	REPS	REPS	REPS
	LOAD	LOAD	LOAD	LOAD	LOAD
	REPS	REPS	REPS	REPS	REPS
	LOAD	LOAD	LOAD	LOAD	LOAD
	REPS	REPS	REPS	REPS	REPS
	LOAD	LOAD	LOAD	LOAD	LOAD
	REPS	REPS	REPS	REPS	REPS
	LOAD	LOAD	LOAD	LOAD	LOAD
	REPS	REPS	REPS	REPS	REPS
	LOAD	LOAD	LOAD	LOAD	LOAD
	REPS	REPS	REPS	REPS	REPS
	LOAD	LOAD	LOAD	LOAD	LOAD
	REPS	REPS	REPS	REPS	REPS
	LOAD	LOAD	LOAD	LOAD	LOAD

CARDIO

NAME / TYPE:				
TIME	**LEVEL**	**DISTANCE**	**HEART RATE**	**CALORIES**

NAME / TYPE:				
TIME	**LEVEL**	**DISTANCE**	**HEART RATE**	**CALORIES**

NOTES / OTHER

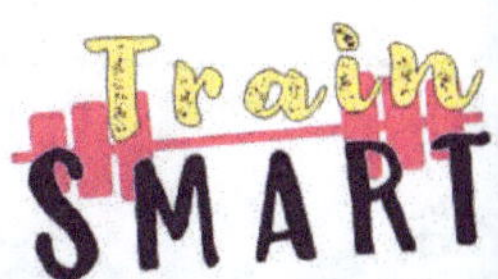

SESSION LOGBOOK

MON	TUE	WED	THU	FRI	SAT	SUN

Date:	Start Time:	Finish Time:

Session Name / Type:

STRENGTH & CONDITIONING

EXERCISE	SET 1	SET 2	SET 3	SET 4	SET 5
	REPS	REPS	REPS	REPS	REPS
	LOAD	LOAD	LOAD	LOAD	LOAD
	REPS	REPS	REPS	REPS	REPS
	LOAD	LOAD	LOAD	LOAD	LOAD
	REPS	REPS	REPS	REPS	REPS
	LOAD	LOAD	LOAD	LOAD	LOAD
	REPS	REPS	REPS	REPS	REPS
	LOAD	LOAD	LOAD	LOAD	LOAD
	REPS	REPS	REPS	REPS	REPS
	LOAD	LOAD	LOAD	LOAD	LOAD
	REPS	REPS	REPS	REPS	REPS
	LOAD	LOAD	LOAD	LOAD	LOAD
	REPS	REPS	REPS	REPS	REPS
	LOAD	LOAD	LOAD	LOAD	LOAD
	REPS	REPS	REPS	REPS	REPS
	LOAD	LOAD	LOAD	LOAD	LOAD
	REPS	REPS	REPS	REPS	REPS
	LOAD	LOAD	LOAD	LOAD	LOAD
	REPS	REPS	REPS	REPS	REPS
	LOAD	LOAD	LOAD	LOAD	LOAD

CARDIO

NAME / TYPE:				
TIME	**LEVEL**	**DISTANCE**	**HEART RATE**	**CALORIES**

NAME / TYPE:				
TIME	**LEVEL**	**DISTANCE**	**HEART RATE**	**CALORIES**

NOTES / OTHER

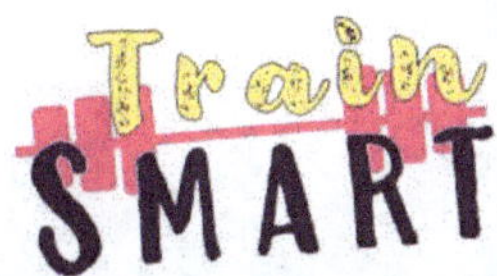

SESSION LOGBOOK

MON	TUE	WED	THU	FRI	SAT	SUN

Date:	Start Time:	Finish Time:

Session Name / Type:

STRENGTH & CONDITIONING

EXERCISE	SET 1	SET 2	SET 3	SET 4	SET 5
	REPS	REPS	REPS	REPS	REPS
	LOAD	LOAD	LOAD	LOAD	LOAD
	REPS	REPS	REPS	REPS	REPS
	LOAD	LOAD	LOAD	LOAD	LOAD
	REPS	REPS	REPS	REPS	REPS
	LOAD	LOAD	LOAD	LOAD	LOAD
	REPS	REPS	REPS	REPS	REPS
	LOAD	LOAD	LOAD	LOAD	LOAD
	REPS	REPS	REPS	REPS	REPS
	LOAD	LOAD	LOAD	LOAD	LOAD
	REPS	REPS	REPS	REPS	REPS
	LOAD	LOAD	LOAD	LOAD	LOAD
	REPS	REPS	REPS	REPS	REPS
	LOAD	LOAD	LOAD	LOAD	LOAD
	REPS	REPS	REPS	REPS	REPS
	LOAD	LOAD	LOAD	LOAD	LOAD
	REPS	REPS	REPS	REPS	REPS
	LOAD	LOAD	LOAD	LOAD	LOAD
	REPS	REPS	REPS	REPS	REPS
	LOAD	LOAD	LOAD	LOAD	LOAD

CARDIO

NAME / TYPE:				
TIME	**LEVEL**	**DISTANCE**	**HEART RATE**	**CALORIES**

NAME / TYPE:				
TIME	**LEVEL**	**DISTANCE**	**HEART RATE**	**CALORIES**

NOTES / OTHER

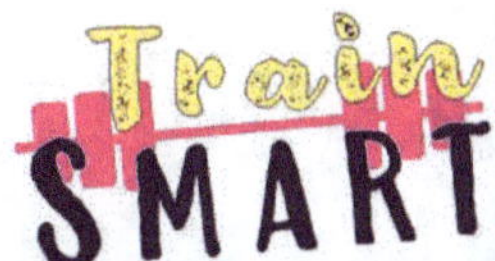

SESSION LOGBOOK

MON	TUE	WED	THU	FRI	SAT	SUN

Date:	Start Time:	Finish Time:

Session Name / Type:

STRENGTH & CONDITIONING

EXERCISE	SET 1	SET 2	SET 3	SET 4	SET 5
	REPS	REPS	REPS	REPS	REPS
	LOAD	LOAD	LOAD	LOAD	LOAD
	REPS	REPS	REPS	REPS	REPS
	LOAD	LOAD	LOAD	LOAD	LOAD
	REPS	REPS	REPS	REPS	REPS
	LOAD	LOAD	LOAD	LOAD	LOAD
	REPS	REPS	REPS	REPS	REPS
	LOAD	LOAD	LOAD	LOAD	LOAD
	REPS	REPS	REPS	REPS	REPS
	LOAD	LOAD	LOAD	LOAD	LOAD
	REPS	REPS	REPS	REPS	REPS
	LOAD	LOAD	LOAD	LOAD	LOAD
	REPS	REPS	REPS	REPS	REPS
	LOAD	LOAD	LOAD	LOAD	LOAD
	REPS	REPS	REPS	REPS	REPS
	LOAD	LOAD	LOAD	LOAD	LOAD
	REPS	REPS	REPS	REPS	REPS
	LOAD	LOAD	LOAD	LOAD	LOAD
	REPS	REPS	REPS	REPS	REPS
	LOAD	LOAD	LOAD	LOAD	LOAD

CARDIO

NAME / TYPE:				
TIME	**LEVEL**	**DISTANCE**	**HEART RATE**	**CALORIES**

NAME / TYPE:				
TIME	**LEVEL**	**DISTANCE**	**HEART RATE**	**CALORIES**

NOTES / OTHER

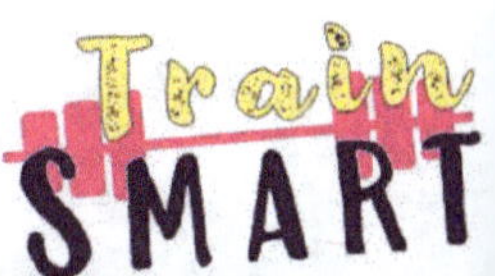

SESSION LOGBOOK

MON	TUE	WED	THU	FRI	SAT	SUN

Date:	Start Time:	Finish Time:

Session Name / Type:

STRENGTH & CONDITIONING

EXERCISE	SET 1	SET 2	SET 3	SET 4	SET 5
	REPS	REPS	REPS	REPS	REPS
	LOAD	LOAD	LOAD	LOAD	LOAD
	REPS	REPS	REPS	REPS	REPS
	LOAD	LOAD	LOAD	LOAD	LOAD
	REPS	REPS	REPS	REPS	REPS
	LOAD	LOAD	LOAD	LOAD	LOAD
	REPS	REPS	REPS	REPS	REPS
	LOAD	LOAD	LOAD	LOAD	LOAD
	REPS	REPS	REPS	REPS	REPS
	LOAD	LOAD	LOAD	LOAD	LOAD
	REPS	REPS	REPS	REPS	REPS
	LOAD	LOAD	LOAD	LOAD	LOAD
	REPS	REPS	REPS	REPS	REPS
	LOAD	LOAD	LOAD	LOAD	LOAD
	REPS	REPS	REPS	REPS	REPS
	LOAD	LOAD	LOAD	LOAD	LOAD
	REPS	REPS	REPS	REPS	REPS
	LOAD	LOAD	LOAD	LOAD	LOAD
	REPS	REPS	REPS	REPS	REPS
	LOAD	LOAD	LOAD	LOAD	LOAD

CARDIO

NAME / TYPE:				
TIME	**LEVEL**	**DISTANCE**	**HEART RATE**	**CALORIES**

NAME / TYPE:				
TIME	**LEVEL**	**DISTANCE**	**HEART RATE**	**CALORIES**

NOTES / OTHER

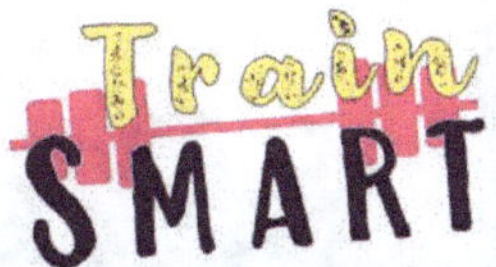

SESSION LOGBOOK

MON	TUE	WED	THU	FRI	SAT	SUN

Date:	Start Time:	Finish Time:

Session Name / Type:

STRENGTH & CONDITIONING

EXERCISE	SET 1	SET 2	SET 3	SET 4	SET 5
	REPS	REPS	REPS	REPS	REPS
	LOAD	LOAD	LOAD	LOAD	LOAD
	REPS	REPS	REPS	REPS	REPS
	LOAD	LOAD	LOAD	LOAD	LOAD
	REPS	REPS	REPS	REPS	REPS
	LOAD	LOAD	LOAD	LOAD	LOAD
	REPS	REPS	REPS	REPS	REPS
	LOAD	LOAD	LOAD	LOAD	LOAD
	REPS	REPS	REPS	REPS	REPS
	LOAD	LOAD	LOAD	LOAD	LOAD
	REPS	REPS	REPS	REPS	REPS
	LOAD	LOAD	LOAD	LOAD	LOAD
	REPS	REPS	REPS	REPS	REPS
	LOAD	LOAD	LOAD	LOAD	LOAD
	REPS	REPS	REPS	REPS	REPS
	LOAD	LOAD	LOAD	LOAD	LOAD
	REPS	REPS	REPS	REPS	REPS
	LOAD	LOAD	LOAD	LOAD	LOAD
	REPS	REPS	REPS	REPS	REPS
	LOAD	LOAD	LOAD	LOAD	LOAD

CARDIO

NAME / TYPE:				
TIME	LEVEL	DISTANCE	HEART RATE	CALORIES

NAME / TYPE:				
TIME	LEVEL	DISTANCE	HEART RATE	CALORIES

NOTES / OTHER

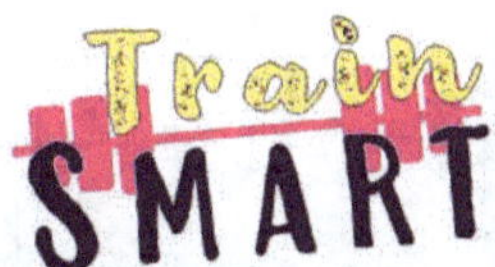

SESSION LOGBOOK

MON	TUE	WED	THU	FRI	SAT	SUN

Date:	Start Time:	Finish Time:

Session Name / Type:

STRENGTH & CONDITIONING

EXERCISE	SET 1	SET 2	SET 3	SET 4	SET 5
	REPS	REPS	REPS	REPS	REPS
	LOAD	LOAD	LOAD	LOAD	LOAD
	REPS	REPS	REPS	REPS	REPS
	LOAD	LOAD	LOAD	LOAD	LOAD
	REPS	REPS	REPS	REPS	REPS
	LOAD	LOAD	LOAD	LOAD	LOAD
	REPS	REPS	REPS	REPS	REPS
	LOAD	LOAD	LOAD	LOAD	LOAD
	REPS	REPS	REPS	REPS	REPS
	LOAD	LOAD	LOAD	LOAD	LOAD
	REPS	REPS	REPS	REPS	REPS
	LOAD	LOAD	LOAD	LOAD	LOAD
	REPS	REPS	REPS	REPS	REPS
	LOAD	LOAD	LOAD	LOAD	LOAD
	REPS	REPS	REPS	REPS	REPS
	LOAD	LOAD	LOAD	LOAD	LOAD
	REPS	REPS	REPS	REPS	REPS
	LOAD	LOAD	LOAD	LOAD	LOAD
	REPS	REPS	REPS	REPS	REPS
	LOAD	LOAD	LOAD	LOAD	LOAD

CARDIO

NAME / TYPE:				
TIME	LEVEL	DISTANCE	HEART RATE	CALORIES

NAME / TYPE:				
TIME	LEVEL	DISTANCE	HEART RATE	CALORIES

NOTES / OTHER

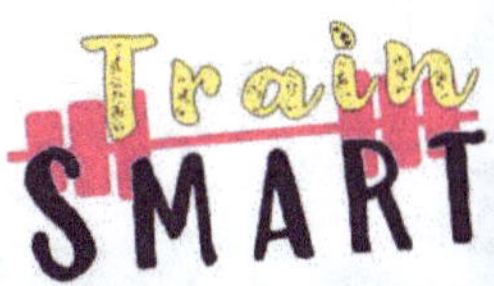

SESSION LOGBOOK

MON	TUE	WED	THU	FRI	SAT	SUN

Date:	Start Time:	Finish Time:

Session Name / Type:

STRENGTH & CONDITIONING

EXERCISE	SET 1	SET 2	SET 3	SET 4	SET 5
	REPS	REPS	REPS	REPS	REPS
	LOAD	LOAD	LOAD	LOAD	LOAD
	REPS	REPS	REPS	REPS	REPS
	LOAD	LOAD	LOAD	LOAD	LOAD
	REPS	REPS	REPS	REPS	REPS
	LOAD	LOAD	LOAD	LOAD	LOAD
	REPS	REPS	REPS	REPS	REPS
	LOAD	LOAD	LOAD	LOAD	LOAD
	REPS	REPS	REPS	REPS	REPS
	LOAD	LOAD	LOAD	LOAD	LOAD
	REPS	REPS	REPS	REPS	REPS
	LOAD	LOAD	LOAD	LOAD	LOAD
	REPS	REPS	REPS	REPS	REPS
	LOAD	LOAD	LOAD	LOAD	LOAD
	REPS	REPS	REPS	REPS	REPS
	LOAD	LOAD	LOAD	LOAD	LOAD
	REPS	REPS	REPS	REPS	REPS
	LOAD	LOAD	LOAD	LOAD	LOAD
	REPS	REPS	REPS	REPS	REPS
	LOAD	LOAD	LOAD	LOAD	LOAD

CARDIO

NAME / TYPE:				

TIME	LEVEL	DISTANCE	HEART RATE	CALORIES

NAME / TYPE:				

TIME	LEVEL	DISTANCE	HEART RATE	CALORIES

NOTES / OTHER

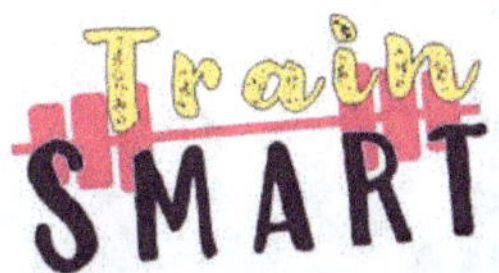

SESSION LOGBOOK

MON	TUE	WED	THU	FRI	SAT	SUN

Date:	Start Time:	Finish Time:

Session Name / Type:

STRENGTH & CONDITIONING

EXERCISE	SET 1	SET 2	SET 3	SET 4	SET 5
	REPS LOAD	REPS LOAD	REPS LOAD	REPS LOAD	REPS LOAD
	REPS LOAD	REPS LOAD	REPS LOAD	REPS LOAD	REPS LOAD
	REPS LOAD	REPS LOAD	REPS LOAD	REPS LOAD	REPS LOAD
	REPS LOAD	REPS LOAD	REPS LOAD	REPS LOAD	REPS LOAD
	REPS LOAD	REPS LOAD	REPS LOAD	REPS LOAD	REPS LOAD
	REPS LOAD	REPS LOAD	REPS LOAD	REPS LOAD	REPS LOAD
	REPS LOAD	REPS LOAD	REPS LOAD	REPS LOAD	REPS LOAD
	REPS LOAD	REPS LOAD	REPS LOAD	REPS LOAD	REPS LOAD
	REPS LOAD	REPS LOAD	REPS LOAD	REPS LOAD	REPS LOAD
	REPS LOAD	REPS LOAD	REPS LOAD	REPS LOAD	REPS LOAD

CARDIO

NAME / TYPE:				
TIME	**LEVEL**	**DISTANCE**	**HEART RATE**	**CALORIES**

NAME / TYPE:				
TIME	**LEVEL**	**DISTANCE**	**HEART RATE**	**CALORIES**

NOTES / OTHER

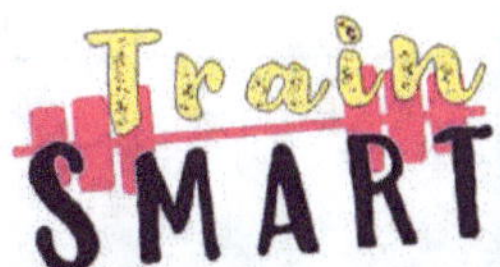

SESSION LOGBOOK

MON	TUE	WED	THU	FRI	SAT	SUN

Date:	Start Time:	Finish Time:

Session Name / Type:

STRENGTH & CONDITIONING

EXERCISE	SET 1	SET 2	SET 3	SET 4	SET 5
	REPS	REPS	REPS	REPS	REPS
	LOAD	LOAD	LOAD	LOAD	LOAD
	REPS	REPS	REPS	REPS	REPS
	LOAD	LOAD	LOAD	LOAD	LOAD
	REPS	REPS	REPS	REPS	REPS
	LOAD	LOAD	LOAD	LOAD	LOAD
	REPS	REPS	REPS	REPS	REPS
	LOAD	LOAD	LOAD	LOAD	LOAD
	REPS	REPS	REPS	REPS	REPS
	LOAD	LOAD	LOAD	LOAD	LOAD
	REPS	REPS	REPS	REPS	REPS
	LOAD	LOAD	LOAD	LOAD	LOAD
	REPS	REPS	REPS	REPS	REPS
	LOAD	LOAD	LOAD	LOAD	LOAD
	REPS	REPS	REPS	REPS	REPS
	LOAD	LOAD	LOAD	LOAD	LOAD
	REPS	REPS	REPS	REPS	REPS
	LOAD	LOAD	LOAD	LOAD	LOAD
	REPS	REPS	REPS	REPS	REPS
	LOAD	LOAD	LOAD	LOAD	LOAD

CARDIO

NAME / TYPE:				
TIME	**LEVEL**	**DISTANCE**	**HEART RATE**	**CALORIES**

NAME / TYPE:				
TIME	**LEVEL**	**DISTANCE**	**HEART RATE**	**CALORIES**

NOTES / OTHER

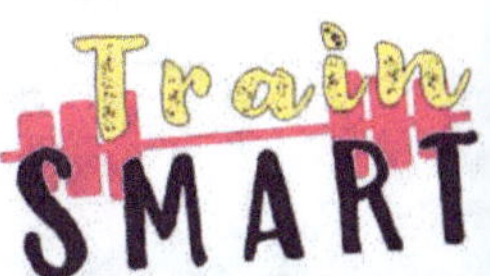

SESSION LOGBOOK

MON	TUE	WED	THU	FRI	SAT	SUN

Date:	Start Time:	Finish Time:

Session Name / Type:

STRENGTH & CONDITIONING

EXERCISE	SET 1	SET 2	SET 3	SET 4	SET 5
	REPS	REPS	REPS	REPS	REPS
	LOAD	LOAD	LOAD	LOAD	LOAD
	REPS	REPS	REPS	REPS	REPS
	LOAD	LOAD	LOAD	LOAD	LOAD
	REPS	REPS	REPS	REPS	REPS
	LOAD	LOAD	LOAD	LOAD	LOAD
	REPS	REPS	REPS	REPS	REPS
	LOAD	LOAD	LOAD	LOAD	LOAD
	REPS	REPS	REPS	REPS	REPS
	LOAD	LOAD	LOAD	LOAD	LOAD
	REPS	REPS	REPS	REPS	REPS
	LOAD	LOAD	LOAD	LOAD	LOAD
	REPS	REPS	REPS	REPS	REPS
	LOAD	LOAD	LOAD	LOAD	LOAD
	REPS	REPS	REPS	REPS	REPS
	LOAD	LOAD	LOAD	LOAD	LOAD
	REPS	REPS	REPS	REPS	REPS
	LOAD	LOAD	LOAD	LOAD	LOAD
	REPS	REPS	REPS	REPS	REPS
	LOAD	LOAD	LOAD	LOAD	LOAD

CARDIO

NAME / TYPE:				
TIME	**LEVEL**	**DISTANCE**	**HEART RATE**	**CALORIES**

NAME / TYPE:				
TIME	**LEVEL**	**DISTANCE**	**HEART RATE**	**CALORIES**

NOTES / OTHER

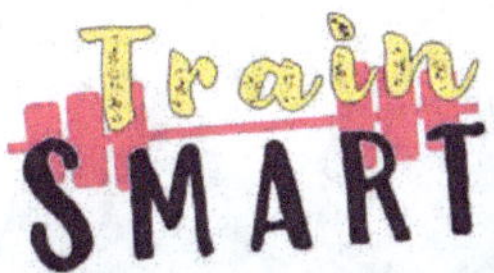

SESSION LOGBOOK

MON	TUE	WED	THU	FRI	SAT	SUN

Date:	Start Time:	Finish Time:

Session Name / Type:

STRENGTH & CONDITIONING

EXERCISE	SET 1	SET 2	SET 3	SET 4	SET 5
	REPS	REPS	REPS	REPS	REPS
	LOAD	LOAD	LOAD	LOAD	LOAD
	REPS	REPS	REPS	REPS	REPS
	LOAD	LOAD	LOAD	LOAD	LOAD
	REPS	REPS	REPS	REPS	REPS
	LOAD	LOAD	LOAD	LOAD	LOAD
	REPS	REPS	REPS	REPS	REPS
	LOAD	LOAD	LOAD	LOAD	LOAD
	REPS	REPS	REPS	REPS	REPS
	LOAD	LOAD	LOAD	LOAD	LOAD
	REPS	REPS	REPS	REPS	REPS
	LOAD	LOAD	LOAD	LOAD	LOAD
	REPS	REPS	REPS	REPS	REPS
	LOAD	LOAD	LOAD	LOAD	LOAD
	REPS	REPS	REPS	REPS	REPS
	LOAD	LOAD	LOAD	LOAD	LOAD
	REPS	REPS	REPS	REPS	REPS
	LOAD	LOAD	LOAD	LOAD	LOAD
	REPS	REPS	REPS	REPS	REPS
	LOAD	LOAD	LOAD	LOAD	LOAD

CARDIO

NAME / TYPE:				
TIME	**LEVEL**	**DISTANCE**	**HEART RATE**	**CALORIES**

NAME / TYPE:				
TIME	**LEVEL**	**DISTANCE**	**HEART RATE**	**CALORIES**

NOTES / OTHER

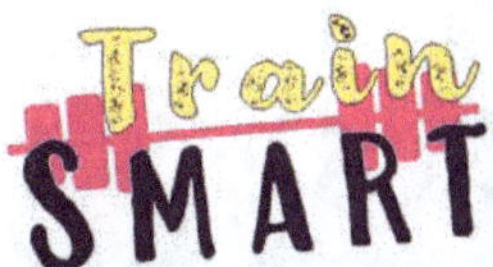

SESSION LOGBOOK

MON	TUE	WED	THU	FRI	SAT	SUN

Date:	Start Time:	Finish Time:

Session Name / Type:

STRENGTH & CONDITIONING

EXERCISE	SET 1	SET 2	SET 3	SET 4	SET 5
	REPS	REPS	REPS	REPS	REPS
	LOAD	LOAD	LOAD	LOAD	LOAD
	REPS	REPS	REPS	REPS	REPS
	LOAD	LOAD	LOAD	LOAD	LOAD
	REPS	REPS	REPS	REPS	REPS
	LOAD	LOAD	LOAD	LOAD	LOAD
	REPS	REPS	REPS	REPS	REPS
	LOAD	LOAD	LOAD	LOAD	LOAD
	REPS	REPS	REPS	REPS	REPS
	LOAD	LOAD	LOAD	LOAD	LOAD
	REPS	REPS	REPS	REPS	REPS
	LOAD	LOAD	LOAD	LOAD	LOAD
	REPS	REPS	REPS	REPS	REPS
	LOAD	LOAD	LOAD	LOAD	LOAD
	REPS	REPS	REPS	REPS	REPS
	LOAD	LOAD	LOAD	LOAD	LOAD
	REPS	REPS	REPS	REPS	REPS
	LOAD	LOAD	LOAD	LOAD	LOAD
	REPS	REPS	REPS	REPS	REPS
	LOAD	LOAD	LOAD	LOAD	LOAD

CARDIO

NAME / TYPE:				
TIME	**LEVEL**	**DISTANCE**	**HEART RATE**	**CALORIES**

NAME / TYPE:				
TIME	**LEVEL**	**DISTANCE**	**HEART RATE**	**CALORIES**

NOTES / OTHER

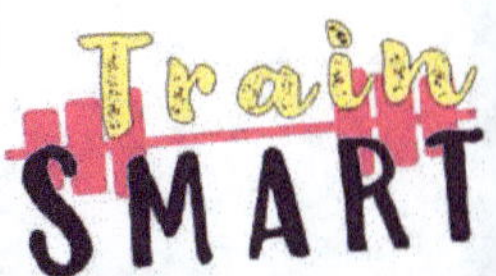

SESSION LOGBOOK

MON	TUE	WED	THU	FRI	SAT	SUN

Date:	Start Time:	Finish Time:

Session Name / Type:

STRENGTH & CONDITIONING

EXERCISE	SET 1	SET 2	SET 3	SET 4	SET 5
	REPS	REPS	REPS	REPS	REPS
	LOAD	LOAD	LOAD	LOAD	LOAD
	REPS	REPS	REPS	REPS	REPS
	LOAD	LOAD	LOAD	LOAD	LOAD
	REPS	REPS	REPS	REPS	REPS
	LOAD	LOAD	LOAD	LOAD	LOAD
	REPS	REPS	REPS	REPS	REPS
	LOAD	LOAD	LOAD	LOAD	LOAD
	REPS	REPS	REPS	REPS	REPS
	LOAD	LOAD	LOAD	LOAD	LOAD
	REPS	REPS	REPS	REPS	REPS
	LOAD	LOAD	LOAD	LOAD	LOAD
	REPS	REPS	REPS	REPS	REPS
	LOAD	LOAD	LOAD	LOAD	LOAD
	REPS	REPS	REPS	REPS	REPS
	LOAD	LOAD	LOAD	LOAD	LOAD
	REPS	REPS	REPS	REPS	REPS
	LOAD	LOAD	LOAD	LOAD	LOAD
	REPS	REPS	REPS	REPS	REPS
	LOAD	LOAD	LOAD	LOAD	LOAD

CARDIO

NAME / TYPE:				
TIME	**LEVEL**	**DISTANCE**	**HEART RATE**	**CALORIES**

NAME / TYPE:				
TIME	**LEVEL**	**DISTANCE**	**HEART RATE**	**CALORIES**

NOTES / OTHER

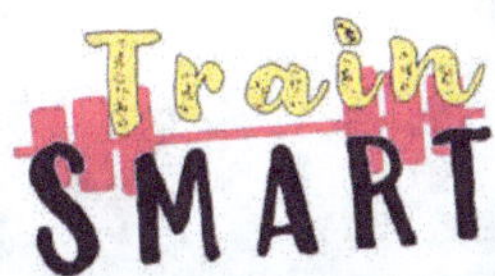

SESSION LOGBOOK

MON	TUE	WED	THU	FRI	SAT	SUN

Date:	Start Time:	Finish Time:

Session Name / Type:

STRENGTH & CONDITIONING

EXERCISE	SET 1	SET 2	SET 3	SET 4	SET 5
	REPS	REPS	REPS	REPS	REPS
	LOAD	LOAD	LOAD	LOAD	LOAD
	REPS	REPS	REPS	REPS	REPS
	LOAD	LOAD	LOAD	LOAD	LOAD
	REPS	REPS	REPS	REPS	REPS
	LOAD	LOAD	LOAD	LOAD	LOAD
	REPS	REPS	REPS	REPS	REPS
	LOAD	LOAD	LOAD	LOAD	LOAD
	REPS	REPS	REPS	REPS	REPS
	LOAD	LOAD	LOAD	LOAD	LOAD
	REPS	REPS	REPS	REPS	REPS
	LOAD	LOAD	LOAD	LOAD	LOAD
	REPS	REPS	REPS	REPS	REPS
	LOAD	LOAD	LOAD	LOAD	LOAD
	REPS	REPS	REPS	REPS	REPS
	LOAD	LOAD	LOAD	LOAD	LOAD
	REPS	REPS	REPS	REPS	REPS
	LOAD	LOAD	LOAD	LOAD	LOAD
	REPS	REPS	REPS	REPS	REPS
	LOAD	LOAD	LOAD	LOAD	LOAD

CARDIO

NAME / TYPE:				
TIME	**LEVEL**	**DISTANCE**	**HEART RATE**	**CALORIES**

NAME / TYPE:				
TIME	**LEVEL**	**DISTANCE**	**HEART RATE**	**CALORIES**

NOTES / OTHER

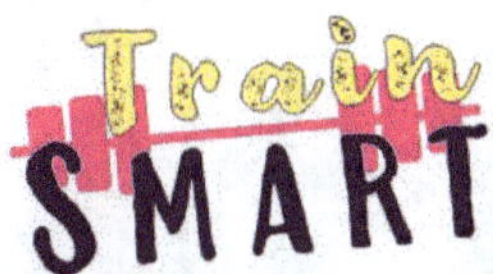

SESSION LOGBOOK

MON	TUE	WED	THU	FRI	SAT	SUN

Date:		Start Time:		Finish Time:	

Session Name / Type:

STRENGTH & CONDITIONING

EXERCISE	SET 1	SET 2	SET 3	SET 4	SET 5
	REPS	REPS	REPS	REPS	REPS
	LOAD	LOAD	LOAD	LOAD	LOAD
	REPS	REPS	REPS	REPS	REPS
	LOAD	LOAD	LOAD	LOAD	LOAD
	REPS	REPS	REPS	REPS	REPS
	LOAD	LOAD	LOAD	LOAD	LOAD
	REPS	REPS	REPS	REPS	REPS
	LOAD	LOAD	LOAD	LOAD	LOAD
	REPS	REPS	REPS	REPS	REPS
	LOAD	LOAD	LOAD	LOAD	LOAD
	REPS	REPS	REPS	REPS	REPS
	LOAD	LOAD	LOAD	LOAD	LOAD
	REPS	REPS	REPS	REPS	REPS
	LOAD	LOAD	LOAD	LOAD	LOAD
	REPS	REPS	REPS	REPS	REPS
	LOAD	LOAD	LOAD	LOAD	LOAD
	REPS	REPS	REPS	REPS	REPS
	LOAD	LOAD	LOAD	LOAD	LOAD
	REPS	REPS	REPS	REPS	REPS
	LOAD	LOAD	LOAD	LOAD	LOAD

CARDIO

NAME / TYPE:				
TIME	LEVEL	DISTANCE	HEART RATE	CALORIES

NAME / TYPE:				
TIME	LEVEL	DISTANCE	HEART RATE	CALORIES

NOTES / OTHER

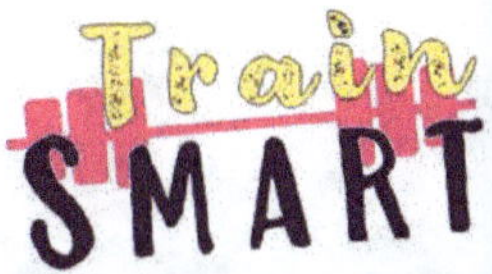

SESSION LOGBOOK

MON	TUE	WED	THU	FRI	SAT	SUN

Date:	Start Time:	Finish Time:

Session Name / Type:

STRENGTH & CONDITIONING

EXERCISE	SET 1	SET 2	SET 3	SET 4	SET 5
	REPS	REPS	REPS	REPS	REPS
	LOAD	LOAD	LOAD	LOAD	LOAD
	REPS	REPS	REPS	REPS	REPS
	LOAD	LOAD	LOAD	LOAD	LOAD
	REPS	REPS	REPS	REPS	REPS
	LOAD	LOAD	LOAD	LOAD	LOAD
	REPS	REPS	REPS	REPS	REPS
	LOAD	LOAD	LOAD	LOAD	LOAD
	REPS	REPS	REPS	REPS	REPS
	LOAD	LOAD	LOAD	LOAD	LOAD
	REPS	REPS	REPS	REPS	REPS
	LOAD	LOAD	LOAD	LOAD	LOAD
	REPS	REPS	REPS	REPS	REPS
	LOAD	LOAD	LOAD	LOAD	LOAD
	REPS	REPS	REPS	REPS	REPS
	LOAD	LOAD	LOAD	LOAD	LOAD
	REPS	REPS	REPS	REPS	REPS
	LOAD	LOAD	LOAD	LOAD	LOAD
	REPS	REPS	REPS	REPS	REPS
	LOAD	LOAD	LOAD	LOAD	LOAD

CARDIO

NAME / TYPE:				
TIME	**LEVEL**	**DISTANCE**	**HEART RATE**	**CALORIES**

NAME / TYPE:				
TIME	**LEVEL**	**DISTANCE**	**HEART RATE**	**CALORIES**

NOTES / OTHER

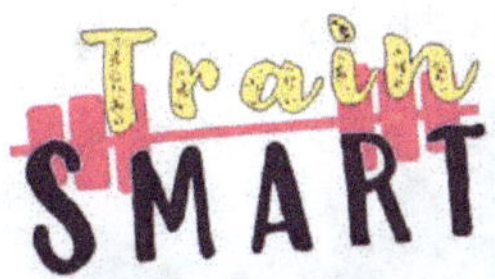

SESSION LOGBOOK

MON	TUE	WED	THU	FRI	SAT	SUN

Date:	Start Time:	Finish Time:

Session Name / Type:

STRENGTH & CONDITIONING

EXERCISE	SET 1	SET 2	SET 3	SET 4	SET 5
	REPS	REPS	REPS	REPS	REPS
	LOAD	LOAD	LOAD	LOAD	LOAD
	REPS	REPS	REPS	REPS	REPS
	LOAD	LOAD	LOAD	LOAD	LOAD
	REPS	REPS	REPS	REPS	REPS
	LOAD	LOAD	LOAD	LOAD	LOAD
	REPS	REPS	REPS	REPS	REPS
	LOAD	LOAD	LOAD	LOAD	LOAD
	REPS	REPS	REPS	REPS	REPS
	LOAD	LOAD	LOAD	LOAD	LOAD
	REPS	REPS	REPS	REPS	REPS
	LOAD	LOAD	LOAD	LOAD	LOAD
	REPS	REPS	REPS	REPS	REPS
	LOAD	LOAD	LOAD	LOAD	LOAD
	REPS	REPS	REPS	REPS	REPS
	LOAD	LOAD	LOAD	LOAD	LOAD
	REPS	REPS	REPS	REPS	REPS
	LOAD	LOAD	LOAD	LOAD	LOAD
	REPS	REPS	REPS	REPS	REPS
	LOAD	LOAD	LOAD	LOAD	LOAD

CARDIO

NAME / TYPE:				
TIME	**LEVEL**	**DISTANCE**	**HEART RATE**	**CALORIES**

NAME / TYPE:				
TIME	**LEVEL**	**DISTANCE**	**HEART RATE**	**CALORIES**

NOTES / OTHER

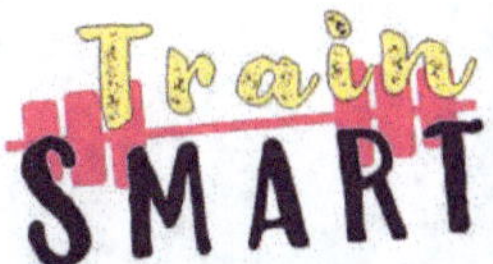

SESSION LOGBOOK

MON	TUE	WED	THU	FRI	SAT	SUN

Date:	Start Time:	Finish Time:

Session Name / Type:

STRENGTH & CONDITIONING

EXERCISE	SET 1	SET 2	SET 3	SET 4	SET 5
	REPS	REPS	REPS	REPS	REPS
	LOAD	LOAD	LOAD	LOAD	LOAD
	REPS	REPS	REPS	REPS	REPS
	LOAD	LOAD	LOAD	LOAD	LOAD
	REPS	REPS	REPS	REPS	REPS
	LOAD	LOAD	LOAD	LOAD	LOAD
	REPS	REPS	REPS	REPS	REPS
	LOAD	LOAD	LOAD	LOAD	LOAD
	REPS	REPS	REPS	REPS	REPS
	LOAD	LOAD	LOAD	LOAD	LOAD
	REPS	REPS	REPS	REPS	REPS
	LOAD	LOAD	LOAD	LOAD	LOAD
	REPS	REPS	REPS	REPS	REPS
	LOAD	LOAD	LOAD	LOAD	LOAD
	REPS	REPS	REPS	REPS	REPS
	LOAD	LOAD	LOAD	LOAD	LOAD
	REPS	REPS	REPS	REPS	REPS
	LOAD	LOAD	LOAD	LOAD	LOAD
	REPS	REPS	REPS	REPS	REPS
	LOAD	LOAD	LOAD	LOAD	LOAD

CARDIO

NAME / TYPE:				
TIME	**LEVEL**	**DISTANCE**	**HEART RATE**	**CALORIES**

NAME / TYPE:				
TIME	**LEVEL**	**DISTANCE**	**HEART RATE**	**CALORIES**

NOTES / OTHER

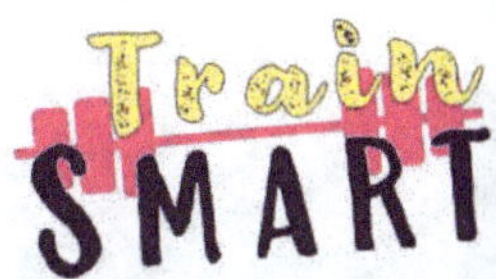

SESSION LOGBOOK

MON	TUE	WED	THU	FRI	SAT	SUN

Date:	Start Time:	Finish Time:

Session Name / Type:

STRENGTH & CONDITIONING

EXERCISE	SET 1	SET 2	SET 3	SET 4	SET 5
	REPS	REPS	REPS	REPS	REPS
	LOAD	LOAD	LOAD	LOAD	LOAD
	REPS	REPS	REPS	REPS	REPS
	LOAD	LOAD	LOAD	LOAD	LOAD
	REPS	REPS	REPS	REPS	REPS
	LOAD	LOAD	LOAD	LOAD	LOAD
	REPS	REPS	REPS	REPS	REPS
	LOAD	LOAD	LOAD	LOAD	LOAD
	REPS	REPS	REPS	REPS	REPS
	LOAD	LOAD	LOAD	LOAD	LOAD
	REPS	REPS	REPS	REPS	REPS
	LOAD	LOAD	LOAD	LOAD	LOAD
	REPS	REPS	REPS	REPS	REPS
	LOAD	LOAD	LOAD	LOAD	LOAD
	REPS	REPS	REPS	REPS	REPS
	LOAD	LOAD	LOAD	LOAD	LOAD
	REPS	REPS	REPS	REPS	REPS
	LOAD	LOAD	LOAD	LOAD	LOAD
	REPS	REPS	REPS	REPS	REPS
	LOAD	LOAD	LOAD	LOAD	LOAD

CARDIO

NAME / TYPE:				
TIME	**LEVEL**	**DISTANCE**	**HEART RATE**	**CALORIES**

NAME / TYPE:				
TIME	**LEVEL**	**DISTANCE**	**HEART RATE**	**CALORIES**

NOTES / OTHER

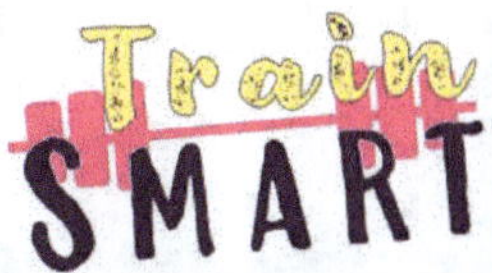

SESSION LOGBOOK

MON	TUE	WED	THU	FRI	SAT	SUN

Date:	Start Time:	Finish Time:

Session Name / Type:

STRENGTH & CONDITIONING

EXERCISE	SET 1	SET 2	SET 3	SET 4	SET 5
	REPS	REPS	REPS	REPS	REPS
	LOAD	LOAD	LOAD	LOAD	LOAD
	REPS	REPS	REPS	REPS	REPS
	LOAD	LOAD	LOAD	LOAD	LOAD
	REPS	REPS	REPS	REPS	REPS
	LOAD	LOAD	LOAD	LOAD	LOAD
	REPS	REPS	REPS	REPS	REPS
	LOAD	LOAD	LOAD	LOAD	LOAD
	REPS	REPS	REPS	REPS	REPS
	LOAD	LOAD	LOAD	LOAD	LOAD
	REPS	REPS	REPS	REPS	REPS
	LOAD	LOAD	LOAD	LOAD	LOAD
	REPS	REPS	REPS	REPS	REPS
	LOAD	LOAD	LOAD	LOAD	LOAD
	REPS	REPS	REPS	REPS	REPS
	LOAD	LOAD	LOAD	LOAD	LOAD
	REPS	REPS	REPS	REPS	REPS
	LOAD	LOAD	LOAD	LOAD	LOAD
	REPS	REPS	REPS	REPS	REPS
	LOAD	LOAD	LOAD	LOAD	LOAD

CARDIO

NAME / TYPE:				
TIME	**LEVEL**	**DISTANCE**	**HEART RATE**	**CALORIES**

NAME / TYPE:				
TIME	**LEVEL**	**DISTANCE**	**HEART RATE**	**CALORIES**

NOTES / OTHER

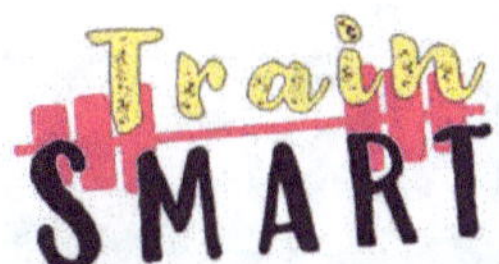

SESSION LOGBOOK

MON	TUE	WED	THU	FRI	SAT	SUN

Date: | Start Time: | Finish Time:

Session Name / Type:

STRENGTH & CONDITIONING

EXERCISE	SET 1	SET 2	SET 3	SET 4	SET 5
	REPS	REPS	REPS	REPS	REPS
	LOAD	LOAD	LOAD	LOAD	LOAD
	REPS	REPS	REPS	REPS	REPS
	LOAD	LOAD	LOAD	LOAD	LOAD
	REPS	REPS	REPS	REPS	REPS
	LOAD	LOAD	LOAD	LOAD	LOAD
	REPS	REPS	REPS	REPS	REPS
	LOAD	LOAD	LOAD	LOAD	LOAD
	REPS	REPS	REPS	REPS	REPS
	LOAD	LOAD	LOAD	LOAD	LOAD
	REPS	REPS	REPS	REPS	REPS
	LOAD	LOAD	LOAD	LOAD	LOAD
	REPS	REPS	REPS	REPS	REPS
	LOAD	LOAD	LOAD	LOAD	LOAD
	REPS	REPS	REPS	REPS	REPS
	LOAD	LOAD	LOAD	LOAD	LOAD
	REPS	REPS	REPS	REPS	REPS
	LOAD	LOAD	LOAD	LOAD	LOAD
	REPS	REPS	REPS	REPS	REPS
	LOAD	LOAD	LOAD	LOAD	LOAD

CARDIO

NAME / TYPE:				
TIME	**LEVEL**	**DISTANCE**	**HEART RATE**	**CALORIES**

NAME / TYPE:				
TIME	**LEVEL**	**DISTANCE**	**HEART RATE**	**CALORIES**

NOTES / OTHER

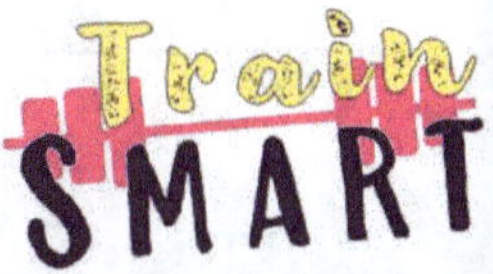

SESSION LOGBOOK

MON	TUE	WED	THU	FRI	SAT	SUN

Date:	Start Time:	Finish Time:

Session Name / Type:

STRENGTH & CONDITIONING

EXERCISE	SET 1	SET 2	SET 3	SET 4	SET 5
	REPS LOAD	REPS LOAD	REPS LOAD	REPS LOAD	REPS LOAD
	REPS LOAD	REPS LOAD	REPS LOAD	REPS LOAD	REPS LOAD
	REPS LOAD	REPS LOAD	REPS LOAD	REPS LOAD	REPS LOAD
	REPS LOAD	REPS LOAD	REPS LOAD	REPS LOAD	REPS LOAD
	REPS LOAD	REPS LOAD	REPS LOAD	REPS LOAD	REPS LOAD
	REPS LOAD	REPS LOAD	REPS LOAD	REPS LOAD	REPS LOAD
	REPS LOAD	REPS LOAD	REPS LOAD	REPS LOAD	REPS LOAD
	REPS LOAD	REPS LOAD	REPS LOAD	REPS LOAD	REPS LOAD
	REPS LOAD	REPS LOAD	REPS LOAD	REPS LOAD	REPS LOAD
	REPS LOAD	REPS LOAD	REPS LOAD	REPS LOAD	REPS LOAD

CARDIO

NAME / TYPE:				
TIME	**LEVEL**	**DISTANCE**	**HEART RATE**	**CALORIES**

NAME / TYPE:				
TIME	**LEVEL**	**DISTANCE**	**HEART RATE**	**CALORIES**

NOTES / OTHER

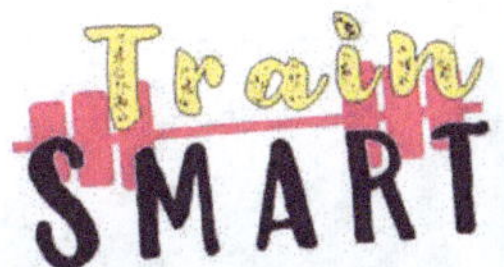

SESSION LOGBOOK

MON	TUE	WED	THU	FRI	SAT	SUN

Date:	Start Time:	Finish Time:

Session Name / Type:

STRENGTH & CONDITIONING

EXERCISE	SET 1	SET 2	SET 3	SET 4	SET 5
	REPS	REPS	REPS	REPS	REPS
	LOAD	LOAD	LOAD	LOAD	LOAD
	REPS	REPS	REPS	REPS	REPS
	LOAD	LOAD	LOAD	LOAD	LOAD
	REPS	REPS	REPS	REPS	REPS
	LOAD	LOAD	LOAD	LOAD	LOAD
	REPS	REPS	REPS	REPS	REPS
	LOAD	LOAD	LOAD	LOAD	LOAD
	REPS	REPS	REPS	REPS	REPS
	LOAD	LOAD	LOAD	LOAD	LOAD
	REPS	REPS	REPS	REPS	REPS
	LOAD	LOAD	LOAD	LOAD	LOAD
	REPS	REPS	REPS	REPS	REPS
	LOAD	LOAD	LOAD	LOAD	LOAD
	REPS	REPS	REPS	REPS	REPS
	LOAD	LOAD	LOAD	LOAD	LOAD
	REPS	REPS	REPS	REPS	REPS
	LOAD	LOAD	LOAD	LOAD	LOAD
	REPS	REPS	REPS	REPS	REPS
	LOAD	LOAD	LOAD	LOAD	LOAD

CARDIO

NAME / TYPE:				
TIME	**LEVEL**	**DISTANCE**	**HEART RATE**	**CALORIES**

NAME / TYPE:				
TIME	**LEVEL**	**DISTANCE**	**HEART RATE**	**CALORIES**

NOTES / OTHER

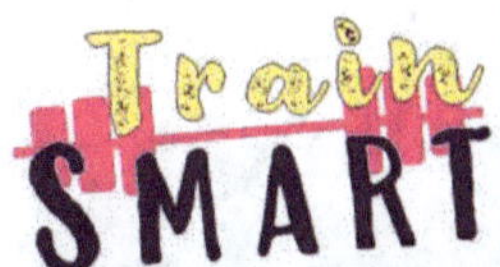

SESSION LOGBOOK

MON	TUE	WED	THU	FRI	SAT	SUN

Date:	Start Time:	Finish Time:

Session Name / Type:

STRENGTH & CONDITIONING

EXERCISE	SET 1	SET 2	SET 3	SET 4	SET 5
	REPS	REPS	REPS	REPS	REPS
	LOAD	LOAD	LOAD	LOAD	LOAD
	REPS	REPS	REPS	REPS	REPS
	LOAD	LOAD	LOAD	LOAD	LOAD
	REPS	REPS	REPS	REPS	REPS
	LOAD	LOAD	LOAD	LOAD	LOAD
	REPS	REPS	REPS	REPS	REPS
	LOAD	LOAD	LOAD	LOAD	LOAD
	REPS	REPS	REPS	REPS	REPS
	LOAD	LOAD	LOAD	LOAD	LOAD
	REPS	REPS	REPS	REPS	REPS
	LOAD	LOAD	LOAD	LOAD	LOAD
	REPS	REPS	REPS	REPS	REPS
	LOAD	LOAD	LOAD	LOAD	LOAD
	REPS	REPS	REPS	REPS	REPS
	LOAD	LOAD	LOAD	LOAD	LOAD
	REPS	REPS	REPS	REPS	REPS
	LOAD	LOAD	LOAD	LOAD	LOAD
	REPS	REPS	REPS	REPS	REPS
	LOAD	LOAD	LOAD	LOAD	LOAD

CARDIO

NAME / TYPE:				
TIME	**LEVEL**	**DISTANCE**	**HEART RATE**	**CALORIES**

NAME / TYPE:				
TIME	**LEVEL**	**DISTANCE**	**HEART RATE**	**CALORIES**

NOTES / OTHER

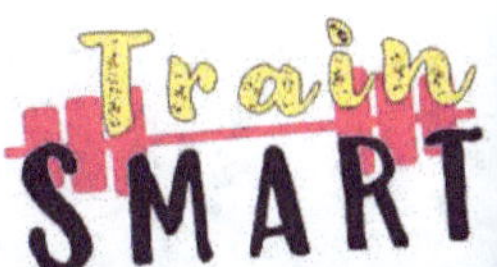

NOTES

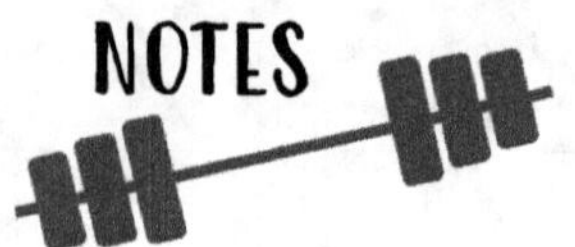

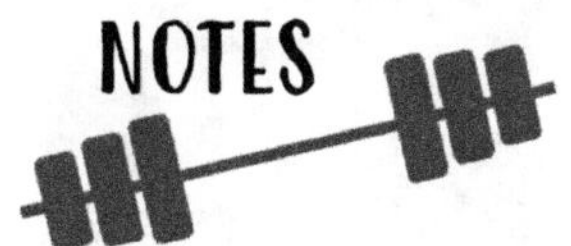

NOTES

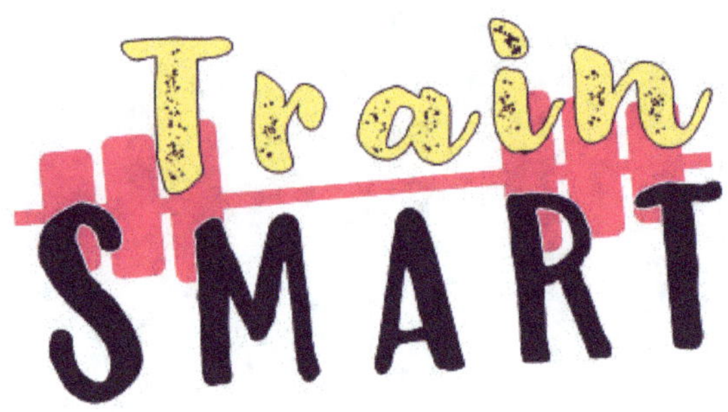

Train Smart Workout Logbook

ISBN: 978-1-9999616-0-2

First published in the UK by Pura Track Publishing in December 2020.

For business enquiries, email: questions@toremathompson.uk

WWW.TOREMATHOMPSON.UK